Review Questions for
PHLEBOTOMY

A Subject Review and Questions for ASCP Phlebotomy Technician Examinations

Dedication

To Ben, Hilary, Jared, Kevin, Rebecca and Stephanie – the next generation

Review Questions for
PHLEBOTOMY

A Subject Review and Questions for ASCP Phlebotomy Technician Examinations

Sara Taylor, MT (ASCP)
University of North Texas Health Science Center
at Fort Worth

Review Questions Series
Series Editor: Thomas R. Gest, PhD
University of Arkansas for Medical Sciences

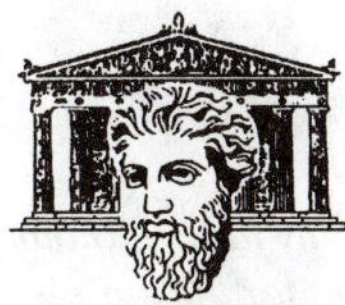

The Parthenon Publishing Group
International Publishers in Medicine, Science & Technology

NEW YORK   LONDON

Published in the USA by
The Parthenon Publishing Group Inc.
One Blue Hill Plaza,
PO Box 1564, Pearl River,
New York 10965, USA

Published in Europe by
The Parthenon Publishing Group Limited
Casterton Hall, Carnforth,
Lancs. LA6 2LA, UK

Copyright © 2000 The Parthenon Publishing Group

Library of Congress Cataloging-in-Publication Data

Taylor, Sara.
  Review questions for phlebotomy : a subject review and questions for ASCP
phlebotomy technician examinations / Sara Taylor.
     p. ; cm. – (Review questions series)
  Includes bibliographical references.
  ISBN 1-85070-755-3 (alk. paper)
  1. Phlebotomy–Examinations, questions, etc.
  [DNLM: I. Phlebotomy–Examination Questions.   WB 18.2 T2471r2000]
  I. Title. II. Title: Phlebotomy. III. Series.
  RB45.15.T39 2000
  616.07′561–dc21

                                 99-044543

British Library Cataloguing in Publication Data

Taylor, Sara.
  Review questions for phlebotomy : a subject review and questions for ASCP
phlebotomy technician examinations. – (Review questions series)
  1. Phlebotomy – Examinations, questions, etc.
  I. Title
  616′.07561′076

ISBN 1-85070-755-3

Printed in the USA

CONTENTS

Numbers in parentheses indicate number of questions available.

ACKNOWLEDGEMENTS

For their generous help in assisting with the editing of this book, I would like to thank the following individuals: Maximilian Borski, BS MS; Lauren Telesca, MT ASCP; Sherry Van Vranken; Don Wager, PhD; and Kathleen Walsh, MT ASCP.

INTRODUCTION

As the complexity of medical technology increases, the profession of phlebotomy or obtaining blood samples from patients grows more complicated as well. Many academic institutions and health organizations have established phlebotomy training courses in order to train individuals in this skilled and technological field. The importance of obtaining and delivering an appropriate specimen sample to the testing laboratory cannot be overemphasized. To help ensure that individuals employed in this field are knowledgeable and competent, increasing numbers of health organizations are requiring that their phlebotomy personnel obtain nationally recognized board certification as a phlebotomy technician.

This review text in phlebotomy is designed to be of assistance to phlebotomists who are preparing for these examinations. In addition to using this book to prepare for one of the board certifying examinations, students may choose to utilize the book to help them prepare for course examinations or for their own performance review. The text is divided into nine sections that between them contain the major content areas of the several national board certifying examinations offered for phlebotomists. The nine sections are as follows:

Section 1.	The phlebotomist's role in the health-care setting
Section 2.	Anatomy and physiology
Section 3.	Infection control and safety
Section 4.	Collection equipment
Section 5.	Collection procedures
Section 6.	Specimen processing (ordering, transport, processing)
Section 7.	Special collections and special handling
Section 8.	Quality control
Section 9.	Interpersonal skills

The book is written in a multiple choice question format. The correct answers are provided along with detailed explanations. In many cases useful information can be provided by having the incorrect choices explained as well, and every attempt was made to do this. At the beginning of each section there is a list of objectives that the ensuing section will cover. Students are encouraged to read the objectives carefully. If after using the questions as a study guide the student feels unsure of his or her knowledge of the objectives, there are numerous commercially available phlebotomy textbooks that should provide helpful explanations. Finally, this text includes a vocabulary list of commonly encountered abbreviations, medical/scientific terms and important prefixes and suffixes.

Board examinations contain questions that are not simply recall questions, but rather contain questions that require an examinee to assimilate several pieces of information. Because this examination style prevails, whenever possible the same types of questions were designed for this review text.

ABBREVIATIONS

ABG	Arterial blood gas. Blood drawn from an artery for determination of blood gases
ABO	Refers to the various types of human blood groups
ADH	Antidiuretic hormone. Also known as vasopressin
AFB	Acid-fast bacillus, the causative agent of tuberculosis
AFP	Alpha-fetoprotein. Levels of this protein help determine neural tube defects in the fetus
A/G	The ratio between the serum proteins albumin and globulin
AIDS	Acronym for acquired immunodeficiency syndrome. The disease manifestation of infection with the HIV virus
Alb	Albumin. A protein. One of the tests included in most chemistry 12 and liver profiles
ALK	See **Alk. Phos**
Alk. Phos	Alkaline phosphatase. An enzyme. One of the tests included in most chemistry 12 and liver profiles. Also known as **ALP** or **ALK**
ALP	See **Alk. Phos**
ALT	Alanine aminotransferase. An enzyme. One of the tests included in most liver profiles. Also known as **SGPT**
Amy	An enzyme. Helps diagnose pancreatic disease
ANA	Antinuclear antibody. A serological test that is performed as a screening test for autoimmune disease
ASAP	As soon as possible
ASCP	American Society of Clinical Pathologists
ASO	Antistreptolysin O titer. Monitors streptococcal exposure
AST	Aspartate aminotransferase. An enzyme. One of the tests included in most chemistry 12 and liver profiles. Also known as **GOT** or **SGOT**
BC	Blood cultures. Blood samples are tested for the presence of bacteria
BC	Birthing center. Expectant mothers give birth in this unit of the hospital
BT	Bleeding time. A test in which a small incision is made on a patient's forearm, and the amount of time the patient requires to stop bleeding is recorded. This test measures platelet function
BUN	Blood urea nitrogen. A non-protein nitrogen compound. One of the tests included in most chemistry 12 profiles
Ca	Calcium. A mineral. One of the tests included in most chemistry 12 profiles
CAP	College of American Pathologists
C&S	Culture and sensitivity. Potentially infectious samples are obtained and swabbed onto agar plates to test for pathogens
CBC	Complete blood count. Performed in the hematology department, CBCs include tests such as WBC and RBC counts, Hgb, Hct and either a manual or automated differential
cc	Cubic centimeter, a milliliter
CCU	Coronary Care Unit
CDC	Center for Disease Control
Chol	Cholesterol. A serum lipid. One of the tests included in most chemistry 12 profiles
Chol/LDL	Cholesterol to low-density lipoprotein ratio. Included in most lipid profiles
Cl	Chloride. An electrolyte. One of the tests included in an electrolyte panel
CLIA	Clinical Laboratory Improvements Act (1988)
CO$_2$	Carbon dioxide. A gas. One of the tests included in an electrolyte panel
Coombs'	Direct Coombs' test. Tests for the presence of antibodies on RBCs
CPK	Creatine phosphokinase. An enzyme. Included in cardiac profile panels
CPR	Cardiopulmonary resuscitation. Rescue method
Cr	Creatinine. A non-protein nitrogen compound. One of the tests included in most chemistry 12 profiles

Cr Cl	Creatinine clearance. A 24-hour test done on urine that evaluates renal function
CRP	C-reactive protein. Found in the serum of persons with active inflammatory conditions
CSF	Cerebral spinal fluid
CQI	Continuous quality improvement
CVC	Central venous catheter
D. Bili	Direct bilirubin. A bile pigment. Total bilirubin minus indirect bilirubin equals direct bilirubin. One of the tests included in most liver profiles. Also known as conjugated bilirubin
Diff	Differential. A smear of blood is viewed under the microscope. The percentages of the several different kinds of WBCs are tallied
DOT	Department of Transportation
EBV	Epstein–Barr virus. A herpesvirus, the probable etiologic agent for infectious mononucleosis
EDTA	Ethylenediaminetetraacetate. The anticoagulant found in lavender-topped vacutainer tubes
EPA	Environmental Protection Agency
ESR	Erythrocyte sedimentation rate. A measure of how far, in millimeters, red blood cells will settle to the bottom of a special graded tube
ER	Emergency Room
ETOH	Alcohol
FBS	Fasting blood sugar. One of the tests for glucose levels in serum. See also **Glu** and **GTT**
FDP	Fibrin degradation products. The products of fibrinolysis
Fe	Iron
FSH	Follicle stimulating hormone. Stimulates follicular growth, ovulation and estrogens
FT$_4$	Free thyrosine. One of the tests used to evaluate thyroid function
GC	Gonorrhea. Infection by the bacteria *Neisseria gonorrhoeae* is determined by a test by this name
GGT	Gamma-glutamyl transferase. An enzyme. One of the tests included in most liver profiles
Glu	Glucose. A carbohydrate, one of the tests included in most chemistry 12 profiles. Also often ordered individually (see **FBS**) or as part of tolerance tests (See **GTT**)
GPT	See **ALT**
GTT	Glucose tolerance test. A test spanning several hours that tests a patient's ability to metabolize a glucose load
H&H	Hemoglobin and hematocrit. Two hematology tests that help diagnose anemia
HAV	Hepatitis A virus
HBV	Hepatitis B virus
Hct	Hematocrit. This is the packed cell volume of blood. If a test tube of blood is centrifuged, the cellular portion, being heavier than the plasma portion, will pack down into the bottom of the test tube
HCV	Hepatitis C virus
HDL	High-density lipoprotein. A type of cholesterol. A test included in most lipid profiles
Hep Bs Ag	Hepatitis B surface antigen
Hgb	Hemoglobin. This measures the amount of hemoglobin, an oxygen-carrying protein in the blood
Hgb A1C	Hemoglobin A1C. Also known as glycosylated hemoglobin. A test used to monitor diabetics' diets
HIV	Human immunodeficiency virus. The causative agent of AIDS
ICU	Intensive Care Unit. The hospital unit reserved for patients in a critical or serious condition
IM	Intramuscular, as in an intramuscular injection
IP	Inorganic phosphorous. Imbalances usually affect calcium levels
IV	Intravenous, in the vein
JCAHO	Joint Commission on the Accreditation of Health Organizations
K	Potassium. An electrolyte. One of the tests included in an electrolyte panel
LDH	Lactate dehydrogenase. An enzyme. One of the tests included in most chemistry 12 and liver profiles
LDL	Low-density lipoprotein. A type of cholesterol. A test included in most lipid profiles
LE prep	Lupus erythematosus preparation. This test helps diagnose a patient with lupus erythematosus, an autoimmune disease

LH	Luteinizing hormone. Stimulates progesterone
LTT	Lactose tolerance test
Lytes	Electrolytes
mg	Milligram, 1/1000 of a gram
Mg	Magnesium. A mineral. A deficiency is associated with muscle and nerve tremors
MLT	Medical laboratory technician. A clinical laboratory professional having an A.S. degree
Mono	Mononucleosis. A serological test that determines the presence of antibodies to the Epstein–Barr virus that causes mononucleosis
MSDS	Material safety data sheet
MT	Medical technologist. A clinical laboratory professional with a B.S. degree
Na	Sodium. An electrolyte. One of the tests included in an electrolyte panel
NBS	National Bureau of Standards
Neobili	Neobilirubin test. A bilirubin test performed on a newborn
NH$_3$	Ammonia. Helpful in diagnosing liver disease
NIDA	National Institute of Drug Abuse
NPO	Nothing per os (by mouth)
Nsy	Nursery. Neonates stay in this hospital unit
OR	Operating Room. The hospital unit designated for surgery
OSHA	Occupational Safety and Health Administration
Pb	Lead
PHS	United States Public Health Service
PKU	Phenylketonuria. This serious and potentially fatal inability to metabolize the amino acid phenylalanine can be tested for with a blood test called a PKU test
Plt	Platelets. One of the cellular constituents of blood
PO$_4$	Phosphate. Phosphate in bones is in the form of $CaPO_4$, levels of one will generally affect the other
PPE	Personal protective equipment
PPG	Postprandial glucose
PSA	Prostatic specific antigen. A diagnostic test for prostate cancer
PT	Protime test. A coagulation test used to monitor coumadin levels
PTT	Partial thromboplastin test. A coagulation test that monitors heparin levels
QNS	Quantity not sufficient. Samples delivered to the laboratory are sometimes in such small amounts that the requested test cannot be performed
RA	Rheumatoid arthritis. Serological test for rheumatoid arthritis
RBC	Red blood cell
Retic	Reticulocyte. A blood smear is made and stained with a special stain that highlights reticulocytes – immature RBCs
RIA	Radioimmunoassay
RPR	The RPR test stands for rapid plasma reagin. It is a serological test for the presence of reagin, an antibody-like substance that results from the interaction of treponema (the causative agent of syphilis) and body tissues
RR	Recovery Room. Patients recover from surgery in this hospital unit
SGOT	See **AST**
SGPT	See **ALT**
SST	Serum-separator tube. A vacutainer tube that contains no anticoagulant, but does contain a gel barrier device that separates red blood cells from serum upon centrifugation
SSU	Short Stay Unit. Patients requiring simple, one-day procedures are cared for in this unit
STAT	From the Latin word 'statim', STAT means 'immediately' or 'at once'
T. Bili	Total bilirubin. A pigment in bile. One of the tests included in most chemistry 12 and liver profiles
T cell	Lymphocyte derived from the thymus. T-cell levels are tracked in HIV-positive patients
TDM	Therapeutic drug monitoring
TIBC	Total iron binding capacity. This test measures the amount of serum transferrin

SECTION 1: THE PHLEBOTOMIST'S ROLE IN THE HEALTH-CARE SETTING

Objectives

- To be able to identify health-care providers and be aware of the phlebotomist's role as a member of the health-care team
- To be able to list and describe the various hospital departments
- To be able to list and describe the various laboratory sections
- To be able to describe laboratory procedures in each laboratory section, and to know what the specimen requirements for each section are
- To be able to describe the organizational structure of the laboratory

Key facts

A. Departments and services within various health-care facilities

    1. Inpatient setting (Hospitals)
        a. Radiology, Diagnostic Imaging (X-Ray)
        b. Nuclear Medicine
        c. Radiation Therapy
        d. Occupational Therapy
        e. Physical Therapy
        f. Respiratory Therapy
        g. Electrocardiography (EKG and EEG)
        h. Pharmacy (in house and outpatient)
        i. Total Quality Management
        j. Clinical Laboratory
        k. Hospital Units
            1. ER
            2. ICU
            3. CCU
            4. OR
            5. RR
            6. BC
            7. Nsy
            8. Med Surg Floors
            9. SSU or Outpatient Surgery
    2. Outpatient facilities
        a. Clinics (primary care, ambulatory patients)
        b. Nursing Homes
        c. Homehealth
        d. HMOs
        e. Group Practices

B. Departments and sections within the Clinical Laboratory, and the types of procedures run in each department

    1. Chemistry
    2. Hematology
    3. Immunohematology (Blood Bank)
    4. Microbiology
    5. Urinalysis
    6. Coagulation
    7. Serology

8. Therapeutic Drug Monitoring
9. Histology, Cytology, Nuclear Medicine

C. Specimen requirements for each laboratory department

D. Organizational chart for clinical laboratory personnel

E. Common medical terminology

Questions and Answers

1.001 Which of the following comprise the common tests of a chemistry 12 profile?

A.	Alb	T. Bili	Ca
	TP	Cr	Uric
	LDH	BUN	Chol
	Glu	AST	
	Alk. Phos		
B.	Na	K	Cl
	CO_2		
C.	Alb	T. Bili	D. Bili
	GGT	AST	LDH
	Alk. Phos	TP	ALT
D.	BUN	Glu	Amy
	IP	Mg	

A. is the correct answer.

B. lists the tests included in an electrolyte panel.
C. lists the tests most often included in a liver profile.
D. is a group of miscellaneous tests.

1.002 Blood drawn for a lead-level determination should be drawn in which of the following vacutubes:
A. Red-topped or SST
B. Lavender-topped or EDTA-preserved
C. Light blue-topped or citrate-preserved
D. Royal blue-topped

D. is the correct answer.

1.003 Blood drawn for Hep Bs Ag should be sent to which laboratory department?
A. Blood Bank
B. Chemistry
C. Hematology
D. Serology

D. is the correct answer.

1.004 Which of the following tests is not performed in the Serological department?
A. RA
B. ESR
C. Hep Bs Ag
D. VDRL

B. is the correct answer.

An ESR is an erythrocyte sedimentation rate. It is done in the Hematology department.
An RA test is a test for rheumatoid arthritis.
The Hep Bs Ag is a test for the envelope protein of the hepatitis B virus.
A VDRL test is a serological test for the antibody-like substance or 'reagin' that results when *Treponema* (the causative agent of syphilis) interacts with body tissues.

1.005   Which of the following tests is not a serological test?
    A. LE prep
    B. ANA
    C. RPR
    D. Rubella

A. is the correct answer.

An LE prep is a lupus erythematosus preparation. This test prepares the buffy coat of blood for microscopic examination of the distinctive cells associated with lupus erythematosus.
An ANA tests for the presence of anti-nuclear antibodies. It is a serological screening test for lupus erythematosus.
The RPR test stands for rapid plasma reagin. It is a serological test for the presence of reagin.
The rubella test is a serological test for the presence of antibodies to the rubella virus.

1.006   Which of the following tests is a serological test?
    A. Mono
    B. PT
    C. PTT
    D. FDP

A. is the correct answer.

This serological test determines the presence of antibodies to the Epstein–Barr virus that causes mononucleosis.
A PT test is a protime test. This coagulation test monitors coumadin levels.
A PTT test is a partial thromboplastin test. It is a coagulation test that monitors heparin levels.
The fibrin degradation products or FDP test is also a coagulation test. It measures amounts of products of fibrinolysis.

1.007   Which of the following are usually collected in a green-stoppered tube?
    A. LE prep (lupus erythematosus prep)
    B. BUN (blood urea nitrogen)
    C. NH_3 (ammonia)
    D. ETOH (alcohol)

A. and C. are correct.

BUN is collected in a red-topped or an SST tube. ETOH is collected in a red-topped or gray-topped tube.

1.008   Which of the following is not collected in a red-topped or SST tube?
    A. TIBC (total iron binding capacity)
    B. Lytes (electrolytes)
    C. CBC (complete blood count)
    D. Reticulocyte

C. and D. are the correct answers.

Both of these tests should be collected in the lavender-topped tube.

1.009   Chemistry tests are usually collected in which vacutainer tube(s)?
    A. Red-topped or SST tube
    B. Lavender-topped tube
    C. Light blue-topped tube
    D. Royal blue-topped tube

A. is the correct answer.

The lavender-topped tube is the tube that most hematology tests are collected in.
The light blue-topped tube is the tube that coagulation tests are collected in.
The royal blue-topped tube is the tube that is used to collect blood that will be analyzed for trace metals.

1.010   Blood collected for a type and screen is delivered to which laboratory department?
A. Hematology
B. Immunohematology (Blood Bank)
C. Serology
D. Microbiology

B. is the correct answer.

1.011   To which laboratory department should blood collected for blood cultures be delivered?
A. Hematology
B. Immunohematology (Blood Bank)
C. Serology
D. Microbiology

D. is the correct answer.

1.012   Which of the following is an alternative name for Dilantin?
A. Carbamazepine
B. Aminophylline
C. Depakene
D. Phenytoin

D. is the correct answer.

The alternative name for carbamazepine is tegretol.
The alternative name for aminophylline is theophylline.
The alternative name for depakene is valproic acid.

1.013   Which of the following is an alternative name for antidiuretic hormone (ADH)?
A. Vasopressin
B. Tricyclic antidepressants
C. Procainamide
D. Lithium

A. is the correct answer.

Tricyclic antidepressants are also known as amitriptyline or nortriptyline.
Procainamide is also known as prontesyl.
Lithium can be used to treat manic depression.

1.014   Which department of the laboratory requires that blood be drawn in a citrate-preserved, light blue-stoppered tube?
A. The Immunohematology (Blood Bank) department
B. The Chemistry department
C. The Coagulation department
D. The Hematology department

C. is the correct answer.

Tests for the Blood Bank should be collected in a plain red-stoppered tube, one without anticoagulants or gel separators.
Most tests in the Chemistry department are collected in an SST or plain red-stoppered tube. Additionally some tests for Chemistry are collected in gray, royal blue, green and lavender-stoppered tubes.
Tests for the Hematology department are generally collected in a lavender-stoppered tube.

1.015   Which of the following chemistry tests are collected in a lavender-stoppered tube?
A. Hemoglobin and hematocrit
B. RBC folate and glycosylated hemoglobin
C. Protime and partial thromboplastin time
D. FDP and fibrinogen

B. is the correct answer.

Hemoglobin and hematocrit tests are collected in a lavender-stoppered tube, but they are hematology tests.
The PT and APTT tests are collected in a light blue-topped tube and are coagulation tests.
The blood for fibrin degradation products (FDP) should be collected in a special light blue-stoppered tube. The blood for fibrinogen should be collected in a regular light blue-stoppered tube.

1.016 Blood drawn for an ETOH level should be sent to which of the following laboratory departments?
A. Blood Bank
B. Chemistry
C. Hematology
D. Microbiology

B. is the correct answer.

1.017 What kind of vacutainer tube should a type and screen be collected in?
A. SST tube
B. Light blue-topped or citrate-preserved tube
C. Plain red-topped tube
D. Lavender-topped or EDTA-preserved

C. is the correct answer.

Serum and red blood cells are utilized in this test. A tube without an anticoagulant is appropriate since serum and not plasma is utilized. A tube with a gel separator is not appropriate since the cells would be contaminated as they were lifted through the gel.

1.018 Cardiac profiles usually include which of the following tests?

A.	Chol	HDL Chol	Trig
	LDL Chol	Chol/LDL Chol (ratio)	
B.	Na	K	CO_2
	Cl		
C.	GOT	CPK	LDH
D.	T_3	T_4	FT_4
	TSH	T_3U	

C. is the correct answer.

A. is a lipid profile.
B. is an electrolyte panel.
D is a thyroid profile.

1.019 In words, this symbol ≥ means:
A. Less than
B. Greater than
C. Greater than or equal to
D. Less than or equal to

C. is the correct answer.

Less than is represented by the symbol <.
Greater than is represented by the symbol >.
Less than or equal to is represented by the symbol ≤.

1.020 Which of the following hospital departments is concerned with the use of radioactive materials to treat disease?
A. Radiology/Diagnostic Imaging
B. Radiation Therapy
C. Occupational Therapy
D. X-ray department

B. is the correct answer.

The Radiology department is concerned with imaging by the use of electromagnetic radiation. Occupational Therapy is adjunctive therapeutic activity for patients.
The X-ray department is now known as Radiology/Diagnostic Imaging.

1.021 Which of the following hospital departments is concerned with graph recordings of the heart's electrical activity?
A. Physical Therapy
B. Respiratory Therapy
C. Electrocardiography
D. Hospice

C. is the correct answer.

The Physical Therapy department uses physical agents such as heat, exercise and electricity for therapeutic purposes.
The department of Respiratory Therapy is concerned with therapeutic activities dealing with breathing.
Hospice units are established for patients in the final stages of a terminal illness.

1.022 Which of the following hospital departments is responsible for analyzing various body fluids and body parts for diagnostic purposes?
A. Pharmacy
B. Total Quality Management
C. Clinical Laboratory
D. Research Laboratory

C. is the correct answer.

The Pharmacy dispenses medicines prescribed by physicians.
The Total Quality Management group or department oversees continuing improvement in the quality of services provided.
Research Laboratories are not directly concerned with clinical care.

1.023 Which of the following laboratory departments test the physical characteristics of blood?
A. Chemistry
B. Hematology
C. Immunohematology (Blood Bank)
D. Microbiology

B. is the correct answer.

The Chemistry department is concerned with testing the chemical constituents of blood such as serum proteins, glucose, lipids, electrolytes, gases, vitamins and enzymes.
The Immunohematology department tests recipients and donors for compatibility with each other so that transfusions of blood and blood products can be administered to patients safely.
The Microbiology department is responsible for the identification of bacterial, viral and fungal pathogens. Microbiology also identifies antibiotics that will be effective against the pathogen.

1.024 Which of the following laboratory departments test antigen–antibody reactions?
A. Urinalysis
B. Coagulation
C. Serology
D. Histology/Cytology

C. is the correct answer.

The Serology department is searching for diseases having an antigen–antibody pathogenesis.
The Urinalysis department performs a variety of tests on urine. The most common of these is the routine urinalysis.
The Coagulation department performs a variety of tests on blood to determine its clotting ability.
The departments of Histology and Cytology examine tissues and cells from surgery, autopsy or biopsy specimens searching for evidence of abnormality.

1.025 In the organizational structure of a hospital, there is a group of people who set hospital policy. This group is known as:
A. The physicians
B. The clinical staff
C. The Board of Directors
D. The TQM group

C. is the correct answer.

Physicians administer to patients.
The clinical staff of a hospital are the health-care professionals that are responsible for the daily testing that is performed in the laboratory. The clinical staff consists of medical technologists, medical laboratory technicians, histotechnologists, cytotechnologists and phlebotomists.
The TQM group oversees continuing improvement in the delivery of services.

1.026 In the organizational structure of a hospital, the person responsible for the day-to-day running of the entire clinical laboratory is:
A. The hospital administrator
B. The laboratory director
C. The laboratory section supervisor
D. The pathologist

B. is the correct answer.

The hospital administrator is the individual who oversees the administration of the policies set by the Board of Directors.
The laboratory section supervisor is responsible for the daily output of the laboratory department of which s/he is in charge.
Although the pathologist is a physician who is in charge of laboratory output, s/he is not concerned with the practical aspects of running the laboratory.

1.027 What type of outpatient facility provides primary care to mostly ambulatory patients who generally do not have a previously scheduled appointment?
A. Walk-in Clinics
B. Nursing Homes
C. Homehealth Agencies
D. Group Practices

A. is the correct answer.

Nursing Homes provide long-term care of patients.
Homehealth Agencies can provide home visits to patients who have a certain amount of independence.
Group Practices are organizations of health-care providers; they may provide services for walk-in patients, but generally like to schedule time for patient visits.

1.028 Which of the following clinical laboratory professionals hold a Bachelor of Science degree?
A. Phlebotomists
B. Medical laboratory technicians
C. Medical technologists
D. Medical assistants

C. is the correct answer.

Bibliography

The American Medical Association Family Medical Guide. New York: Random House, 1987

Dox I, Melloni B, Eisner G. *Melloni's Illustrated Medical Dictionary*. 3rd edn. Carnforth, UK: Parthenon Publishing, 1993

Tortora G, Grabowski S. *Principles of Anatomy and Physiology*. 8th edn. New York, NY: Harper Collins College Publishers, 1996

Pendergraph G. *Handbook of Phlebotomy*. 3rd edn. Philadelphia, London: Lea and Febiger, 1992

Garza D, Becan-McBride K. *Phlebotomy Handbook*. 3rd edn. Norwalk, CT: Appleton and Lange, 1993

NCCLS Specimen Collection. *Procedures for the Collection of Diagnostic Blood Specimens by Venipuncture*. NCCLS Document H3-A3, Vol. 11, No. 10, July 1991

SECTION 2:   ANATOMY AND PHYSIOLOGY

Objectives

- To describe the ten main body systems
- To describe the functions of the main body systems
- To describe the exchange of gases during respiration
- To describe the major constituents of the blood
- To describe the general coagulation process
- To describe the role of the clinical laboratory in assessing body systems

Key facts

A.   Structure and function of the ten main body systems:
1. Skeletal
2. Muscular
3. Nervous
4. Respiratory
5. Digestive
6. Reproductive
7. Endocrine
8. Urinary
9. Integumentary
10. Circulatory
    a. Method and function of the circulatory system
    b. Blood components
        1. WBC
        2. RBC
        3. Platelets
        4. Non-cellular components (plasma and serum)
    c. Coagulation

Questions and Answers

2.001   Which of the following are the smallest of blood vessels, the vessels through which gas, nutrient and waste exchange occurs?
A. Arteries
B. Veins
C. Capillaries
D. None of the above

C. is the correct answer.

Blood exits the heart through the largest-diameter arteries of the body, the aorta and the pulmonary trunk. These arteries branch into smaller arteries, eventually becoming yet smaller arterioles, and then finally becoming the smallest vessels of all – the capillaries. After blood leaves the capillaries, it enters small-diameter venules which merge into larger veins, finally emptying into the largest veins of all – the superior and inferior vena cava.

2.002   Which of the following best describes the heart?
A. It is a double pump
B. There are three circulatory paths so it is a triple pump
C. It has four chambers, it is a quadruple pump
D. None of the above

A. is the correct answer.

The heart has a left side consisting of two chambers that is responsible for systemic circulation and a right side, also consisting of two chambers, that is responsible for pulmonary circulation. These two sides make the heart a double pump. Although the heart has four chambers, two of the chambers work together on the same side.

2.003   Blood that leaves the left ventricle via the aorta and after completing its circulatory circuit returns to the right atrium has traveled which circuit?
A. The systemic circuit
B. The pulmonary circuit
C. The coronary circuit
D. None of the above

A. and C. are the correct answers.

The coronary artery branches off the aorta and supplies the heart wall with blood, so it is actually part of the systemic circuit.
The pulmonary circuit begins when blood leaves the right ventricle and ends when the blood returns to the heart in the left atrium.

2.004   Which of the following describes the pulmonary circuit?
A. Blood leaves the left ventricle, enters the aorta, travels to the periphery of the body and returns to the right atrium
B. Blood leaves the left ventricle, enters the aorta, enters the coronary artery, travels to the heart wall and then returns to the right atrium
C. Blood leaves the right ventricle, enters the pulmonary trunk, travels to the lungs and then returns to the left atrium
D. None of the above

C. is the correct answer.

A. is a description of the systemic circuit.
B. is a description of a special part of the systemic circuit, the coronary circulatory path.

2.005 Which of the following are the chamber(s) of the heart that receive blood from other parts of the body?
A. Left atrium
B. Left ventricle
C. Right atrium
D. Right ventricle

A. and C. are the correct answers.

The atria are the chambers of the heart that receive blood either from the periphery of the body excluding the lungs (right atrium), or from the lungs (left atrium). The ventricles are the pumping chambers of the heart. They receive blood from the atria and then pump it either to the periphery of the body excluding the lungs (left ventricle) or to the lungs (right ventricle).

2.006 Which are the blood vessels that carry blood away from the heart?
A. Veins
B. Arteries
C. Arterioles
D. Capillaries

B. and C. are the correct answers.

Arteries carry blood away from the heart. Arterioles are small-diameter arteries. Veins carry blood back towards the heart. Capillaries are the smallest-diameter blood vessels that are in the tissues of the body. They are exchange sites. At the capillaries, there is an exchange of gases, nutrients and waste products between the tissue cells and the capillary blood.

2.007 Which valve prevents backflow of blood into the left ventricle?
A. Pulmonary semilunar
B. Tricuspid
C. Bicuspid (mitral)
D. Aortic semilunar

D. is the correct answer.

The aortic semilunar valve is a one-way 'door' that allows blood to leave the left ventricle, and prevents its return.
The pulmonary semilunar prevents backflow of blood into the right ventricle.
The tricuspid valve allows blood into the right ventricle but prevents it from backflowing into the right atrium.
The bicuspid or the mitral valve prevents the backflow of blood from the left ventricle into the left atrium.

2.008 Which blood vessels have valves associated with them?
A. Capillaries
B. Arteries
C. Veins
D. None of the above

C. is the correct answer.

Veins have valves distributed along their length. The purpose of these valves is to prevent backflow of blood. The arteries have the strong pumping action of the heart behind them, and so have no need of valves. Capillaries are exchange sites for nutrients, gases and waste products.

2.009 Which of the following contains the innermost layer of the pericardium as well as the outermost layer of the heart wall?
A. Fibrous pericardium
B. Serous pericardium
C. Myocardium
D. Endocardium

B. is the correct answer.

The pericardium is the membrane that covers the heart. It has several layers. The outermost layer is called the fibrous pericardium, the inner layer is the serous pericardium. The serous pericardium has two layers. The outer layer is called the outer parietal; this folds inwards to become the inner visceral or epicardium. This epicardium is the innermost layer of the pericardium as well as the outermost layer of the heart wall.
The endocardium is the innermost layer of the heart wall.

2.010 The endocardium is continuous with:
A. The valves of the heart
B. The epithelial lining of the blood vessels
C. The pericardium
D. None of the above

B. is the correct answer.

The endocardium is a very smooth layer of the heart wall composed of simple squamous epithelium. It is smooth so that there are no rough surfaces that may initiate blood clotting. It is continuous with the smooth epithelial lining of the blood vessels, for uninterrupted smoothness.

2.011 Where is the mitral (bicuspid) valve located?
A. Between the right atrium and the right ventricle
B. At the base of the pulmonary trunk
C. Between the left atrium and the left ventricle
D. At the base of the aorta

C. is the correct answer.

The tricuspid valve is between the right atrium and the right ventricle.
The pulmonary semilunar valve is at the base of the pulmonary trunk.
The aortic semilunar valve is at the base of the aorta.

2.012 In a blood pressure reading, the number that reflects the height that a column of mercury can be raised by the pressure inside the arteries when the ventricle is contracting is:
A. The top number of a reading, the diastolic number
B. The top number of a reading, the systolic number
C. The bottom number of a reading, the diastolic number
D. The bottom number of a reading, the systolic number

B. is the correct answer.

When the ventricles are contracting, they are said to be undergoing systole. When the ventricles are relaxed, they are undergoing diastole. The top number of a blood pressure reading is the systolic, or ventricular systolic number. The bottom number of a blood pressure reading is the diastolic number. It refers to the height that mercury in a column can be raised by the pressure inside the arteries when the ventricle is relaxed.

2.013 Which of the following is a normal heart rate?
A. Approximately 72 beats/minute
B. Approximately 50 beats/minute
C. Approximately 18 beats/minute
D. Approximately 100 beats/minute

A. is the correct answer.

2.014 Which of the following is stroke volume?
    A. The actual amount of blood pumped by the left ventricle
    B. The actual amount of blood pumped by the right ventricle
    C. The amount of blood that circulates throughout the body in 1 minute
    D. Stroke volume × normal heart rate

A. is the correct answer.

The amount of blood that circulates throughout the body in 1 minute is known as the cardiac output. It can be determined by multiplying the stroke volume × normal heart rate.

2.015 Which of the following tests might be done in order to obtain information about the skeletal system?
    A. Uric acid test
    B. Erythrocyte sedimentation rate (ESR)
    C. Rheumatoid arthritis test (RA)
    D. Thyroid tests (T_3, T_4, FT_4, TSH and T_3U)

A., B., C. and D. are the correct answers.

Increased uric acid levels indicate gout, which is a type of arthritis.
Damage to joints can result in arthritis, which can cause an increased ESR.
Damage to joints can result in arthritis, which can cause a positive RA test.
Thyroid tests are considered to be tests of the endocrine system, but abnormalities of the endocrine system can result in giantism or dwarfism, which greatly affect the skeletal system.

2.016 Which of the following tests might be done in order to obtain information about the skeletal system?
    A. Calcium (Ca) test
    B. Phosphate (PO_4) test
    C. Alkaline phosphatase (Alk. Phos, ALP, ALK) test
    D. None of the above

A., B. and C. are all correct.

Low calcium levels can mean that bone stores of calcium are low; increased calcium is found in certain bone diseases.
Phosphate is closely tied to calcium levels, most PO_4 in bones is in the form of $CaPO_4$ and imbalances in the metabolism of either will generally affect the other.
Increased levels of alkaline phosphatase are found in bone cancer. However, increased levels are normal in growing individuals.

2.017 Which of the following tests will not yield any information about the muscular system?
    A. CPK
    B. LDH
    C. GOT
    D. TP

D. is the correct answer.

CPK, LDH and GOT are all cardiac enzymes. The heart is composed of cardiac muscle.

2.018 Epinephrine, norepinephrine, dopamine and acetylcholine are all:
    A. Liver function tests
    B. Neurotransmitters
    C. Kidney function tests
    D. Drugs

B. is the correct answer.

2.019   Many tests of the chem 12 profile assess liver function. Elevations in which of the following chem 12 profile tests may cause the clinician to order a liver profile?
A. Na, K, Cl and CO_2
B. CPK, LDH and GOT
C. LDH, T. Bili, ALP, SGOT, Alb, TP and Chol
D. Glu, BUN, CR, Uric and Ca

C. is the correct answer.

A. These are the tests of the electrolyte panel.
B. These are the tests of the cardiac profile. CPK is not one of the tests in a liver profile.
D. These are tests of the chem 12 profile, but not the ones that would alert a clinician to a liver problem.

2.020   The liver profile is a profile of tests specifically aimed at assessing liver function. The tests included in a liver profile are:

A.	Alb	T. Bili	Ca
	TP	Cr	Uric
	LDH	BUN	Chol
	Glu	AST	
	Alk. Phos		
B.	Na	K	Cl
	CO_2		
C.	Alb	T. Bili	D. Bili
	GGT	AST	LDH
	Alk. Phos	TP	ALT
D.	None of the above		

C. is the correct answer.

A. lists the tests most often included in a chem 12 profile.
B. lists the tests included in an electrolyte panel.

2.021   In addition to the liver profile test, what other laboratory test is a liver function test?
A. CO_2
B. BUN
C. Hep Bs Ag
D. NH_3

D. is the correct answer.

2.022   Since the liver is part of the digestive system, liver profiles help diagnose problems with the digestive system. Which of the following tests are additional tests of the digestive system?
A. Amylase and lipase
B. BUN and CR
C. UA and UC
D. Creatinine clearance

A. is the correct answer.

Amylase and lipase can help diagnose acute and chronic pancreatitis, respectively. The pancreas is part of the digestive system.
B. Blood urea nitrogen (BUN) and creatinine (CR) are tests that assess kidney function.
C. Urinalysis (UA) and urine culture (UC) are also tests of the urinary system.
D. The 24-hour creatinine clearance test also is a test of the urinary system.

2.023   Which of the following would not be helpful in assessing the reproductive system?
A. Testosterone
B. Progesterone and estrogen
C. LH
D. LDH

D. is the correct answer.

LDH is lactate dehydrogenase – an enzyme not associated with the reproductive system.
Testosterone is the male sex hormone.
Progesterone and estrogen are female sex hormones.
LH is an abbreviation for luteinizing hormone which stimulates progesterone.

2.024 Which of the following would not be helpful in assessing the reproductive system?
A. Prolactin
B. FSH
C. Semen analysis
D. Genital cultures

There are no correct answers.

Prolactin stimulates mammary tissue in preparation for breast feeding.
Follicle stimulating hormone (FSH) stimulates follicular growth, ovulation and estrogens.
A semen analysis is a male fertility analysis.
Genital cultures help identify genital pathogens and their sensitivity to antibiotics.

2.025 Which of the following tests would be of no help in assessing the respiratory system?
A. Aminophylline
B. Blood gases
C. Vasopressin
D. Theophylline

C. is the correct answer.

Vasopressin is another name for antidiuretic hormone (ADH).
Aminophylline is a drug used to treat asthma.
Blood gases include the gases exchanged by the respiratory system, O_2 and CO_2.
Theophylline is another name for aminophylline which is a bronchodilator.

2.026 Which of the following depicts the correct sequence of events in the clotting process?
A. Prothrombin activator converts prothrombin to thrombin, which converts fibrinogen to fibrin
B. Prothrombin activator converts thrombin to prothrombin, which converts fibrinogen to fibrin
C. Prothrombin activator converts prothrombin to thrombin, which converts fibrin to fibrinogen
D. None of the above

A. is the correct answer.

2.027 The difference between plasma and serum is that:
A. Serum contains fibrinogen, plasma does not
B. Plasma contains fibrin, serum does not
C. Plasma contains fibrinogen, serum does not
D. There is no difference between plasma and serum

C. is the correct answer.

2.028 The cellular portion of blood includes all of the following except:
A. WBCs
B. RBCs
C. Platelets
D. Plasma

D. is the correct answer.

2.029 The function of the WBCs is primarily:
A. To carry oxygen
B. To initiate the clotting process
C. To fight infection
D. They have no known function

C. is the correct answer

It is the function of the RBCs to carry oxygen.
It is the function of the platelets to initiate the clotting process.

2.030 Which of the following is a granulocyte:
A. Monocyte
B. Lymphocyte
C. Neutrophil
D. Platelet

C. is the correct answer.

2.031   Which are the WBCs that produce antibodies?
    A. Monocytes
    B. Lymphocytes
    C. Neutrophils
    D. Platelets

B. is the correct answer.

Monocytes have a phagocytic and immune response function.
The neutrophils have a phagocytic function.
The function of the platelets is to initiate clotting.

Bibliography

ALBA's Medical Technology. 9th edn. Board Examination Review. Anaheim, CA: A Berkeley Scientific Publication, 1951

Dox I, Melloni B, Eisner G. *Melloni's Illustrated Medical Dictionary*. 3rd edn. Carnforth, UK: Parthenon Publishing, 1993

Tortora G, Grabowski S. *Principles of Anatomy and Physiology*. 8th edn. New York, NY: Harper Collins College Publishers, 1996

Marieb E. *Human Anatomy and Physiology*. 3rd edn. Redwood City, CA: The Benjamin/Cummings Publishing Company, 1995

Van Wynsberghe D, Noback CR, Carola R. *Human Anatomy and Physiology*. 3rd edn. New York, NY: McGraw-Hill, 1995

Garza D, Becan-McBride K. *Phlebotomy Handbook*. 3rd edn. Norwalk, CT: Appleton and Lange, 1993

NCCLS Specimen Collection. *Procedure for the Collection of Diagnostic Blood Specimens by Venipuncture*. NCCLS Document H3-A3, Vol. 11, No. 10, July 1991

SECTION 3: INFECTION CONTROL AND SAFETY

Objectives

- To describe basic programs for infection control
- To describe proper techniques for handwashing, gowning, gloving, masking, entering and exiting isolation rooms
- To describe proper techniques for clean up of spills and decontamination
- To describe isolation procedures
- To describe routes of infection and intervention
- To identify and properly label biohazardous material

Key facts

A.   Transmission routes of infection
1.   Direct contact
    a.   Percutaneous
    b.   Non-intact skin
2.   Indirect contact
3.   Fecal–oral
4.   Airborne

B.   Infection control program
1.   Surveillance (see Section 1)
2.   Hepatitis
3.   AIDS
4.   Isolation
    a.   Complete
    b.   Wound and skin
    c.   Respiratory
    d.   Enteric
    e.   Reverse
5.   Infection control
    a.   Reducing nosocomial infection
        1.   Specific isolation techniques (handwashing, masking, gowning, gloving)
        2.   Entering and exiting isolation rooms
        3.   Biohazard bags for transport
        4.   Good techniques for phlebotomists
6.   Protection techniques (universal precautions)
    a.   Handwashing
    b.   Barrier protection
        1.   Gloves
        2.   Shields
        3.   Masks
        4.   Lab coats
    c.   Injury prevention (see Section 4)
    d.   Waste disposal
        1.   Biohazardous
        2.   Sharps

C.   Cleansing and sanitation of workplace
1.   Levels of sanitation
2.   Decontamination of spills

D.   Electrical safety

E.   Fire safety

F.   Mechanical safety

G.   Chemical safety

Questions and Answers

3.001   The percutaneous route of transmission is a type of:
   A. Direct transmission
   B. Indirect transmission
   C. Airborne transmission
   D. Fecal–oral route

A. is the correct answer.

The transmission routes of infection are outlined as follows:
   Direct contact
      percutaneous
      non-intact skin
   Indirect contact
   Fecal–oral route
   Airborne transmission.

3.002   Sprays, splatter, droplet formation, aerosols and splashing of infectious material are all examples of:
   A. Fecal–oral route of infection
   B. Airborne transmission
   C. Carelessness
   D. Etiologic agents

B. is the correct answer.

The fecal–oral route of infection involves transmission of the pathogen from infected fecal material to the gastrointestinal tract of the potential host.

3.003   Which of the following protective equipment is necessary in order to prevent airborne transmission of infectious material?
   A. Gowns and gloves only
   B. Gowns, gloves and surgical masks
   C. Gowns, gloves and full facial protection such as shields
   D. Personal respirators

C. is the correct answer.

Because airborne transmission of pathogens usually involves pathogen transfer to the potential host across mucous membranes, masks, eye protection and/or face shields should be worn. Gowns and gloves made of or lined with a material that inhibits permeability of infectious material should also be worn.
Personal respirators should be worn whenever there is a risk of aerosolized *Mycobacterium tuberculosis*.

3.004   A laboratory worker sneezes into his hand and then handles some laboratory equipment. A few minutes later, a co-worker touches this same equipment and then wipes her eyes. This is an example of transfer of infectious material by:
   A. Direct contact
   B. Indirect contact
   C. Contact potential
   D. Contagion

B. is the correct answer.

Direct contact refers to the transfer of infectious material from one infectious agent to the next potential host without any intermediate steps, e.g. needlesticks or via mucous membranes.

3.005   The process of monitoring the control of infection in a clinical institution to ensure that the spread of infections falls within the minimally acceptable range is known as:
   A. Evaluation
   B. Monitoring
   C. Surveillance
   D. Observation

C. is the correct answer.

If the occurrences of infection are deemed to be outside the minimally acceptable range, then the institution should have some methodology in place to correct the situation. (See Section 9, questions 9.017 and 9.018 regarding JCAHO's 10-Step Process of the Monitoring and Evaluation Process.)

3.006   Which of the following is one of the most effective barriers to infection?
   A. A cotton laboratory coat
   B. Surgical scrubs
   C. Eyeglasses
   D. Intact skin

D. is the correct answer.

Laboratory coats should be made of materials that resist spatter penetration (not cotton). The coats should also cover the front of the wearer completely, and have long sleeves that completely cover the arms.
Most surgical scrubs do not have long sleeves. Eyeglasses do not prevent splatter from the sides.

3.007   Which of the following viruses might be transmitted to a laboratory worker through a bloody feces sample?
   A. HIV (human immunodeficiency virus)
   B. HBV (hepatitis B virus)
   C. HCV (hepatitis C virus)
   D. HAV (hepatitis A virus)

A., B., C. and D. are all correct.

HIV is transmitted through various body fluids; blood is especially implicated in its transfer.
HBV is commonly known as 'serum hepatitis'. One of the primary modes of transmission is felt to be via direct or indirect contact with blood and blood products.
HCV can be transmitted via blood or blood products, as well as enterically (fecal–oral route).
HAV is transmitted enterically.

3.008   A phlebotomist entering the room of a patient who is in reverse isolation should take which of the following precautions?
   A. A patient in reverse isolation is not infectious to others – no special precautions are necessary
   B. Phlebotomist should wash hands and check to see if donning mask, gloves and gown are indicated
   C. Phlebotomist should wash hands, don gown and gloves, and wear a personal respirator
   D. Phlebotomists should not enter the rooms of patients in reverse isolation

B. is the correct answer.

A patient in reverse isolation is not infectious to others but this person has a weakened immune system and is endangered by the bacteria that the general population is capable of fighting off. People in reverse isolation need to be protected from infection.

3.009   Which of the following precautions should be taken when entering the room of a patient who is in complete isolation?
   A. Isolation bags for specimen transport should be left just outside the room
   B. Phlebotomist should wash hands and then don gloves, mask and gown before entering
   C. Only take the supplies that are needed into the room. Regularly used reusable supplies should be left in an isolation room
   D. All of the above

D. is the correct answer.

3.010 Which of the following precautions need to be taken when exiting the room of a patient who is in complete isolation?
A. All supplies taken into the room with the exception of the blood supply should be disposed of in the room
B. Gloved hands should be washed in the room and the faucet turned off with a paper towel
C. Near the inside of the door, contaminated clothing should be removed by turning inside out and placed in a receptacle
D. After exiting, hands should be washed once again before proceeding to the next patient

A., B., C. and D. are all correct.

3.011 Patients with postoperative wounds, infected catheters and intravenous devices are often placed in what kind of isolation?
A. Wound and skin isolation
B. Respiratory isolation
C. Complete isolation
D. Enteric isolation

A. is the correct answer.

Respiratory isolation is for patients with diseases communicable by airborne transmission. Complete isolation is for patients with serious contagious diseases that may be transmitted by direct contact and by airborne transmission. Patients infected with pathogens that are transmitted by the fecal–oral route may be placed in enteric isolation.

3.012 Which of the following is not a general precaution that should be taken by phlebotomists when procuring blood samples?
A. Discard needles or lancets that have been used for an unsuccessful blood draw
B. Decontaminate skin in venipuncture area
C. Once the cover has been removed from lancets or needles, be sure that they only come in contact with clean areas prior to use
D. Inspect needles and lancets prior to use, checking for spurs or barbs

C. is the correct answer.

Once the cover has been removed from lancets or needles, they should not come in contact with anything before they are used.

3.013 A health-care worker should gown, glove and mask when entering the room of a patient in:
A. Enteric isolation
B. Complete isolation
C. Respiratory isolation
D. Reverse isolation

B., C. and D. are all correct.

Generally, when a patient is in enteric isolation, workers do not need to mask since the pathogens involved are spread by contact with the alimentary canal or by contact with products of the alimentary canal.
Personal respirators should be worn whenever there is a risk of aerosolized *Mycobacterium tuberculosis*.

3.014 The plastic collar that surrounds the rubber stopper of many vacutainer tubes is called a 'hemaguard'. Its purpose is to:
A. Make the tubes easier to grip
B. Prevent aerosols upon stopper removal
C. Allow today's sophisticated instruments to process without human intervention
D. Color code the vacutainers

B. is the correct answer.

3.015 If a tube does not have a hemaguard, if the stopper is removed, it should be:
   A. Covered with an impenetrable material and the stopper should be pulled off towards the handler
   B. Covered with an impenetrable material and the stopper should be pulled off away from the handler
   C. Not removed, the contents should be evacuated into a syringe
   D. Discarded

A. is the correct answer.

The top of the stopper should be pulled off towards the person opening the tube, while avoiding pointing the stopper bottom towards others. In this way, the contaminated bottom will flip out away from the handler.

3.016 One of the recommendations published by the Center for Disease Control is that the blood and body fluid precautions should be used consistently for all patients. This is known as:
   A. JCAHO's 10-Step Process of the Monitoring and Evaluation Process
   B. Total Quality Management
   C. Universal Precautions
   D. OSHA's Infection Control Program

C. is the correct answer.

JCAHO's 10-Step Process of the Monitoring and Evaluation Process pertain to continuous quality improvement which is more thoroughly covered in Section 9.
Total Quality Management refers to continually improving output, covered more thoroughly in Section 9.
OSHA's Infection Control Program is more thoroughly covered in question 3.021 below.

3.017 Under which of the following conditions is it not necessary for a health-care worker to wash his/her hands?
   A. Whenever there is visible contamination
   B. Upon arrival at work
   C. In between each patient contact and before initial patient contact
   D. Before leaving the laboratory

B. is the correct answer.

In addition to A., C. and D., it would be appropriate for health-care workers to wash their hands before engaging in any activities that might bring contaminated hands into contact with mucous membranes and after removing gloves.

3.018 Proper handwashing technique includes:
   A. Placing paper towels on a nearby non-contaminated surface prior to handwashing
   B. Washing once to remove gross contamination, rinsing and washing again to clean fingernails
   C. Turning the water off prior to drying hands
   D. Disposing of the paper towel and then exiting the bathroom

A. and B. are the correct answers.

Hands should be dried, and then the water should be turned off, using the paper towel.
The bathroom should be exited, utilizing a paper towel to protect from contamination from the inside door handle and the towel should be disposed of outside the bathroom.

3.019 In what order should a gown, gloves and mask be donned?
   A. Gloves, mask and then gown
   B. Mask, gloves and then gown
   C. Gloves, gown and then mask
   D. Gown, mask and then gloves

D. is the correct answer.

3.020 How often should latex gloves be changed?
   A. Only when they develop tears
   B. Between patient contacts, whenever there is visible contamination, whenever there may be physical or chemical deterioration, and periodically
   C. Every 20 minutes
   D. Once a day

B. is the correct answer.

3.021   OSHA recommends that all institutions employing people who are at risk of being exposed to infectious disease have an oral and written policy of specific procedures designed to limit exposure to infectious disease. This policy is known as:

A. OSHA's 10-Step Process of the Monitoring and Evaluation Process
B. OSHA's Total Quality Management
C. OSHA's Universal Precautions
D. OSHA's Infection Control Program

D. is the correct answer.

3.022   What are OSHA's recommendations concerning disinfectants used for decontaminating work surfaces after there has been a spill involving potentially infectious material?

A. A solution of 5.25% sodium hypochlorite (household bleach) be used to flood the area
B. A solution of 5.25% sodium hypochlorite (household bleach) diluted between 1:10 and 1:100 be used to flood the area
C. A solution of 10% sodium hypochlorite be used to flood the area
D. A solution of 100% sodium hypochlorite be used to flood the area

B. is the correct answer.

3.023   The procedure that kills pathogenic micro-organisms and their spores is known as:

A. Disinfection
B. Antisepsis
C. Sterilization
D. Sepsis

C. is the correct answer.

Disinfecting procedures kill pathogenic organisms but not necessarily their spores. Disinfectants are used on non-living surfaces.
Antiseptics are cleansing agents that are used on skin; they will reduce the numbers of bacteria on skin.

3.024   How does OSHA recommend that contaminated needles be disposed of?

A. Needles should be bent, recapped or sheared and then placed in a puncture-proof container
B. Needles should not be bent, recapped, sheared or removed from the blood-drawing device by hand. They should be placed in a puncture-proof container labeled as biohazardous
C. They should be incinerated
D. None of the above

B. and C. are the correct answers.

After B has been attended to, the needles should be incinerated.

3.025   Most masks become ineffective after approximately how many minutes of wear?

A. 8 hours
B. 5 minutes
C. 15 minutes
D. 20 minutes

D. is the correct answer.

3.026   Which of the following objects should be disposed of in a biohazard bag?

A. Lancets
B. Capillary tubes
C. Microscope slides and coverslips
D. Bloody gauze

D. is the correct answer.

Biohazard bags are soft-sided containers and should not be used for any medical waste that is a sharp or has the potential to break and become a sharp.

3.027   Which of the following is not a regulatory agency whose regulations must be complied with when disposing of medical waste?
A. Local ordinances
B. State and Federal EPA regulations
C. State and Federal OSHA regulations
D. CDC regulations

D. is the correct answer.

The regulations of local ordinances, State and Federal EPA regulations and State and Federal OSHA regulations should all be met when disposing of medical waste. The CDC offers recommendations but no regulations that must be adhered to.

3.028   The use of steam heat under pressure to achieve sterilization is known as:
A. Incineration
B. Autoclaving
C. Boiling
D. Antisepsis

B. is the correct answer.

Incineration is burning.
Boiling does not involve the use of pressure.
Antisepsis inhibits the action of micro-organisms.

3.029   In order for sterilization to be achieved, micro-organisms and their spores must be destroyed. What are 'spores'?
A. Fungi associated with micro-organisms
B. Hard capsules containing a micro-organism's reproductive material
C. Eggs
D. Anaerobic bacteria

B. is the correct answer.

Spores are much more difficult to destroy than the micro-organism itself. If a micro-organism's spores survive, they may be able to become viable organisms.

3.030   Fires that involve materials that are normally combustible such as paper, wood, plastics and cloth are classified as:
A. Class A fires
B. Class B fires
C. Class C fires
D. Class D fires

A. is the correct answer.

Class B fires involve flammable liquids such as gasoline, solvents, oils and paint.
Class C fires occur in conjunction with electrical equipment.
Class D fires occur in conjunction with combustible metals.

3.031   What kind of fire extinguisher contains dry chemicals and can be used on any type of fire?
A. Class A extinguishers
B. Class B extinguishers
C. Class C extinguishers
D. Multipurpose or ABC extinguishers

D. is the correct answer.

Class A extinguishers are either dry chemical or pressurized water. A water-filled extinguisher should never be used on a Class B or C fire.
Class B extinguishers are filled with foam, dry chemical or carbon dioxide.
Class C extinguishers are filled with either dry chemical or carbon dioxide.

3.032   Which regulatory agency provides the guidelines that a laboratory should adhere to concerning electrical, fire, mechanical and chemical safety of its employees?
A. CDC. The Center for Disease Control
B. CAP. College of American Pathologists
C. JCAHO. The Joint Commission on the Accreditation of Healthcare Organizations
D. OSHA. Occupational Safety and Health Administration

D. is the correct answer.

The Center for Disease Control. This agency makes recommendations concerning disease control.
The College of American Pathologists. One of the governing agencies that can provide accreditation for a clinical laboratory.
The Joint Commission of the Accreditation of Healthcare Organizations is another governing agency that can provide accreditation for a clinical laboratory.

3.033   The information sheets that must be on file for each chemical kept in the laboratory are called:
A. PPE sheets
B. MSDS sheets
C. Safety Manual
D. Procedure Manual

B. is the correct answer.

PPE is an acronym for 'personal protective equipment'. PPE includes such items as laboratory coats, shields, masks, gloves and fume hoods.
The Safety Manual is a document in the clinical laboratory that elaborates all the safety practices of the lab. It must be up-to-date and reviewed regularly by personnel.

3.034   Which of the following information is not included in an MSDS sheet?
A. Hazardous ingredients
B. Fire and explosion hazards
C. First aid procedures
D. Educational inservices about the chemical

D. is the correct answer.

Educational inservices should be held regularly as part of the laboratory's attention to safety.

3.035   When a biohazardous spill occurs in the laboratory, which is the correct order of cleanup?
A. Sweep up any sharps with stiff cardboard, apply household bleach to the spill, apply detergent to spill, absorb and dispose of
B. Sweep up any sharps with stiff cardboard, apply household bleach to spill, absorb with cat litter and dispose of, apply detergent to spill, absorb with cat litter and dispose of
C. Sweep up any sharps with stiff cardboard, absorb spill with cat litter and dispose of, apply detergent to spill, absorb with cat litter and dispose of, apply household bleach to spill, absorb and dispose of
D. Apply household bleach only, then wipe up with disposable towels

C. is the correct answer.

The purpose of absorbing the spill before the disinfectant is that blood contains protein which can inactivate or lessen the activity of the disinfectant. Applying the detergent before the disinfectant provides a dilution effect and also removes interfering proteins.

3.036   If a chemical is splashed into the eye, what is the recommended minimum amount of time that the eye should be rinsed with water?
A. 5 minutes
B. 10 minutes
C. 15 minutes
D. 20 minutes

C. is the correct answer.

3.037   An infection that is acquired in the hospital is called a(n) _________________ infection.
A. Parenteral
B. Indirect
C. Nosocomial
D. Direct

C. is the correct answer.

Parenteral inoculation refers to an inoculation of infectious blood that was not through the alimentary tract. For phlebotomists, basically this means a needlestick inoculation.

3.038   Since many people at home utilize sharps such as lancets and needles to provide home health-care for themselves, how can these people safely dispose of their contaminated sharps?
   A. They should place their sharps in a puncture-proof container and dispose of with their regular waste
   B. They should place their sharps in a puncture-proof container and then incinerate
   C. The contaminated sharps must be contained in a puncture-proof container and then these containers are to given to a health-care institution that will dispose of the waste in a manner consistent with their own policies of disposal
   D. People with contaminated sharps at home should not attempt to dispose of them themselves. Upon proper notification, the State will send someone to collect them

C. is the correct answer.

It is now State law in many States that health-care institutions such as hospitals and nursing homes accept contaminated sharps from the public on certain days of the month.

3.039   Which of the following are precautions that should be taken when working around electrical equipment?
   A. Be sure that the equipment and its electrical cords and power switches are in good repair
   B. Employees should know the locations of circuit breaker boxes
   C. Employees should know that if a dangerous situation involving electricity develops, that the electrical power supply should be cut, either at the breaker box or by pulling the plug (if this can be done safely)
   D. All of the above

D. is the correct answer.

Bibliography

Marx JF. Understanding the varieties of viral hepatitis. *Nursing* 1998;28:43–9

NCCLS Specimen Collection. *Protection of Laboratory Workers from Infectious Disease Transmitted by Blood, Body Fluids, and Tissue*. NCCLS Document M29-T2, Vol. 11, No. 14, September 1991

NCCLS Specimen Collection. *Procedures for the Collection of Diagnostic Blood Specimens by Venipuncture*. Vol. 11, No. 10, July 1991

Garza D, Becan-McBride K. *Phlebotomy Handbook*. 3rd edn. Norwalk, CT: Appleton and Lange, 1993

Rules and Regulations. *Federal Register* 1991;56:No. 235, December 6

Little LM, Murad JL. Guide to safety in the workplace: occupational exposure to hazardous chemicals in laboratories. *Clin Lab Sci* 1993;6:79–81

Hepatitis C. http://marge.metrokc.gov/health/prevcoat/hepcpam.htm

What is Hepatitis? http://www.gep-help.com/generic/hepliv/whatshep.htm

Needles, lancets accepted. *Press and Sun Bulletin*. July 20, 1996. Binghamton, NY

Fox Hospital takes needles, lancets. *Press and Sun Bulletin*. July 21, 1996. Binghamton, NY

http://www.vbg.org/FIRE/Fire-ext.htm

SECTION 4: COLLECTION EQUIPMENT

Objectives

- To ID the various tubes used in the evacuated tube system and the anticoagulants contained therein.
- To discuss the action and importance of various anticoagulants
- To ID the supplies used in an evacuated tube draw
- To ID the supplies used in a syringe draw
- To ID the supplies used in a skin puncture
- Knowledge of the correct order of draw in the various methods of draw
- To ID the supplies used in neonatal blood collection
- To ID the supplies used in arterial blood gas collection
- To ID the supplies used in capillary blood gas collection

Key facts

A. Equipment for venipuncture
    1. Tourniquets
    2. Cleansing solutions
    3. Sterile gauze pads
    4. Bandages
    5. Needles
        a. Gauge
        b. Multidraw
        c. Single draw
        d. Leur adapters
        e. Butterflies
    6. Vacuum tubes
        a. Additives
            1. SST
            2. No additive
            3. STAT
            4. Oxalates
            5. Citrates
            6. EDTA
            7. Heparin
            8. Na fluoride
            9. Thymol (FDP tubes)
        b. Needle holder
        c. Size (pediatric, standard)
    7. Syringes
        a. Indications for use (see Section 5)
        b. Components
    8. Sharps containers

B. Equipment for skin puncture
    1. Small-bore capillary tubes
    2. Large-bore capillary tubes
    3. Unopette system
    4. Microcontainers
    5. Lancets
    6. Autolets

C.   Equipment for arterial blood gas collection (see Section 7)
1.   Heparinized syringes
2.   Needles
3.   Ice

D.   Equipment for capillary blood gas collection
1.   Natelson tubes
2.   Fleas

Questions and Answers

4.001   What is the maximum length of time that a tourniquet should be applied prior to the venipuncture?
    A. The time should not exceed 1–2 minutes
    B. The time should not exceed 1 minute
    C. The time should not exceed 5 minutes
    D. The time should not exceed 20 minutes

A. is the correct answer.

Generally speaking, the time that a tourniquet is applied should not exceed 1–2 minutes, although many sources limit the application time to 1 minute.

4.002   A tourniquet that is applied too long before the venipuncture may cause:
    A. Hemoglobin
    B. Hemoconcentration
    C. Fibrinolysis
    D. Hemolysis

B. is the correct answer.

Hemoconcentration is an increase in certain substances in the blood such as proteins, potassium, cholesterol, coagulation factors and blood cells.
Hemoglobin is a protein that is part of RBCs that carries oxygen.
Fibrinolysis is the degradation of a blood clot and hemolysis is the rupturing of RBCs.

4.003   Which of the following is a suitable cleansing solution for preparing a site for venipunture?
    A. Sterile alcohol prep pads
    B. Povidone-iodine-based prep pads or sticks
    C. Soap and water
    D. All of the above

D. is the correct answer.

Alcohol and iodine are the more commonly used cleansing agents in preparing a venipuncture site. Although not routinely used, soap and water are very effective.

4.004   Which of the following is considered good technique when cleansing a site for venipuncture?
    A. Wipe once with a quick upwards swipe
    B. Wipe once with a quick downwards swipe
    C. Begin cleansing at the point of intended venipuncture, cleanse outwards in concentric circles
    D. Scrub hard in an up and down direction to help raise the vein

C. is the correct answer.

It is felt that bacteria get physically pushed away from the venipuncture site if this technique is used. There is some thought that the alcohol prep pads that are so commonly used do not provide much antibacterial effect, and that pushing the bacteria away from the venipuncture site is their only useful purpose.

4.005   Which of the following needles would be the best choice for a venipuncture on a patient with fragile veins?
    A. A 21-gauge needle
    B. A 23-gauge needle
    C. A 25-gauge needle
    D. An 18-gauge needle

B. is the best answer.

Gauge refers to the diameter of the needle. The smaller the number, the larger the diameter of the needle. 21- and 22-gauge needles are most commonly used for obtaining blood samples. Smaller-gauge needles may be used on pediatric patients and patients with small, fragile veins, but the smaller the gauge, the more the blood is traumatized. In this case, a 25-gauge needle is probably too small to use for blood collection.

4.006   What is a multidraw needle?
   A. The type of needle that is used in the vacutube system
   B. A single needle that is held in a plastic needle holder and is used to collect several tubes of blood
   C. A needle that is sharp on both ends
   D. The type of needle that is used in the syringe system of blood collection

A., B. and C. are the correct answers.

The needle is held in the middle of the needle holder, the end of the needle used for venipuncture extends freely, and the opposite point of the needle is within the cylinder of the holder. This end of the needle is covered with a flexible rubber sheath. The sheath is pushed up and out of the way when a vacuum tube is pushed onto the needle. The sheath comes down and covers the point of the needle when the tube is removed, and in this way prevents blood leakage out of the needle when changing tubes.

4.007   What is a single-draw needle?
   A. The needle that is used in a syringe assembly
   B. A needle with only a single sharp end, the other end screws into the end of the syringe barrel
   C. The needle that is used in the vacutainer system of blood collection
   D. There is no such needle

A. and B. are correct answers.

Unlike the multidraw needle, it only has a single sharp end for insertion into the patient's vein. The other end either locks with a partial twist or screws onto the end of the syringe barrel. All the blood that is to be collected is drawn into the syringe barrel. It will then need to be distributed among appropriate vacuum tubes.

4.008   What is a Leur adapter?
   A. A (usually small-gauge) needle outfitted with plastic tabs on either side of its base, making it easy to hold in place
   B. A plastic collar that covers vacutainer stoppers
   C. A device that fits onto the end of a needle and the tip of the syringe barrel, making incompatible needles and syringes compatible
   D. None of the above

C. is the correct answer.

A. is the description of a butterfly needle.
B. is the description of a hemaguard.

4.009   Under what circumstances might a phlebotomist rather use a butterfly needle than the vacutainer system?
   A. When drawing ambulatory patients
   B. When drawing patients with small or fragile veins
   C. When drawing patients for blood donation
   D. When drawing patients for more than one test

B. is the correct answer.

Typically, the gauges on butterflies are 23 or 25. These small needles are less likely to damage tiny or fragile veins. Secondly, butterflies can adapt to either a syringe or a pediatric tube holder, thereby lessening the amount of vacuum that is exerted on the patient's vein.
Because butterflies can reduce the damage and lessen the likelihood of collapsing tiny and/or fragile veins, they are often preferred for pediatric, geriatric, oncology (cancer) and burn patients.

4.010 What is an SST tube?
    A. A serum separator tube
    B. A tube with a gel barrier
    C. A tube with no additives
    D. A tube that clots the blood STAT

A. and B. are the correct answers.

The SST tube contains an inert gel that has a specific gravity intermediate between the specific gravity of clotted blood and the specific gravity of serum. Upon centrifugation, the RBCs and fibrin clot will be on the bottom of the tube, the serum will be on the top, and the gel separator will position itself between the clot and the serum, creating a physical barrier between them.

4.011 Which is the tube that has no additive?
    A. An SST tube
    B. An orange/black camouflage (STAT) tube
    C. a red-topped tube
    D. A royal blue-topped tube

C. is the correct answer.

The additive of an SST tube is the gel barrier. Orange and black camouflage-stoppered tubes contain tiny glass particles or silicon dust that increase the speed of clotting by mixing with the blood and activating the clotting mechanism.

4.012 What type of anticoagulant is used in gray-stoppered tubes?
    A. EDTA
    B. Potassium oxalate and sodium fluoride or sodium fluoride and thymol
    C. Sodium citrate
    D. No anticoagulant

B. is the correct answer.

4.013 Which of the following tubes is a good choice to use for a STAT glucose test?
    A. An SST tube
    B. A red-topped tube
    C. A gray-stoppered tube
    D. A light blue-stoppered tube

C. is the correct answer.

The anticoagulants of the gray-stoppered tubes act as glycolytic inhibitors. After blood has been removed from the body, the cells continue to metabolize. In the course of cell metabolism, glucose gets broken down (lysed) into smaller components. Glycolytic inhibitors reduce the amount of glucose that gets broken down into smaller subunits; therefore, the glucose results are not falsely depressed when this anticoagulant is used.

4.014 What is the anticoagulant in a light blue-stoppered tube?
    A. EDTA
    B. Sodium citrate
    C. Fluoride
    D. No anticoagulant

B. is the correct answer.

4.015 Which of the following tests need to be collected in a sodium citrate tube?
    A. CBC
    B. Most chemistry tests
    C. PTs and PTTs
    D. FDPs

C. is the correct answer.

Another common coagulation test that requires blood drawn in a light blue-stoppered tube is the FDP test.

4.016 Green-stoppered vacutainer tubes contain a variety of anticoagulants. What chemical do they all have in common?
A. Fluoride
B. Oxalate
C. Thymol
D. Heparin

D. is the correct answer.

Green-stoppered tubes may contain sodium heparin, lithium heparin or ammonium heparin. The chemical common to all of them is heparin. This anticoagulant works by inhibiting thrombin, a blood protein that is essential for clotting. Without this necessary component of clotting, the blood remains as cells and plasma.

4.017 Why is EDTA a good anticoagulant for hematology testing?
A. It facilitates accurate platelet counts and accurate differential readings
B. It allows for quick turn-around time
C. It lyses the RBCs
D. It makes the hemoglobin easy to visualize

A. is the correct answer.

EDTA prevents platelet aggregation, allowing for an accurate count.
Differentials involve smearing a thin layer of blood on a slide and viewing it under the microscope. EDTA-preserved blood will undergo a minimum of distortion of the cellular elements when being made into a smear for microscopic observation.

4.018 In what way does a phlebotomist collect a specimen for a manual differential?
A. The phlebotomist never needs to collect a specimen for a manual differential, this is done by the technologist in the laboratory
B. The phlebotomist makes a thin smear of blood on a microscope slide to be used in performing the manual differential
C. Manual differentials are no longer done
D. Manual differentials are not performed on patient samples

B. is the correct answer.

To perform a differential, a thin layer of blood is smeared across a microscope slide and then stained to facilitate viewing. The several different types of WBCs are counted and tallied so that after 100 cells are counted, a percentage of each type of WBC is known. The RBCs are observed for morphological features, but are not counted.

4.019 Immunohematology, or blood banking, is concerned with providing compatible donated blood to recipients. What kind of tube is used to collect blood for most blood bank tests?
A. A plain red-topped tube
B. An SST tube
C. Either a plain red-topped or an SST tube
D. Neither the plain red-topped nor the SST tube

A. is the correct answer.

In an SST tube, the gel separator will position itself between the clot and the serum, creating a physical barrier between them. In blood bank testing, the laboratory tests the patient's serum, searching for proteins called antibodies. The patient's red blood cells are also tested for antigens, proteins that reside on the surface of the cells. Since this gel separator limits access to the red blood cells, and because red blood cells are needed for blood bank testing, an SST tube would not be an appropriate choice.

4.020   Since it is permissible to collect blood to be used for potassium levels in a green-topped tube, why is it not permissible to use this tube for collecting blood to have electrolyte testing?
A. It is permissible
B. Because green-topped tubes always contain heparin, and this will degrade sodium, falsely lowering the sodium results
C. Because green-stoppered tubes may contain sodium heparin as an anticoagulant and this will falsely elevate sodium readings
D. They are expensive and should be used with discretion

C. is the correct answer.

4.021   What is the anticoagulant used in the light blue-stoppered tubes used for coagulation tests?
A. Sodium heparin
B. Sodium citrate
C. Sodium fluoride
D. Thymol

B. is the correct answer.

4.022   Which of the following tubes should be used to collect blood to be used for therapeutic drug testing?
A. A plain red-topped tube
B. An SST tube
C. Either a plain red-topped or an SST tube
D. Neither a plain red-topped nor an SST tube

A. is the correct answer.

The SST tube contains an inert polymer gel that has a specific gravity intermediate between the specific gravity of red blood cells and the specific gravity of serum. This means that upon centrifugation, it will migrate in between these two blood components, creating a physical barrier between them. However, it is believed that the gel absorbs some of the drug from the serum, falsely lowering the results.

4.023   Which of the following should not be used for collecting blood to be used for general chemistry testing?
A. Orange and black camouflage tubes
B. Red and black camouflage tubes
C. Plain red-topped tubes
D. Gray-topped tubes

D. is the correct answer.

Gray-topped tubes should not be used for general chemistry testing because gray-topped tubes usually contain some type of fluoride anticoagulant, either potassium oxalate and sodium fluoride or sodium fluoride and thymol. General chemistry profiles contain enzyme tests which will be destroyed by fluoride.

4.024   Which of the following tubes are not used to collect blood for blood bank testing?
A. Plain red-topped tubes
B. Lavender-topped tubes
C. Red and black camouflage tubes
D. Orange and black camouflage tubes

C. and D. are the correct answers.

Red and black camouflage tubes are SST tubes. Refer to question 4.019 for an explanation of why this tube is unsuitable for blood bank work. Orange and black camouflage tubes contain tiny glass particles or silicon dust that increase the speed of clotting by mixing with the blood and activating the clotting mechanism. These particles will become trapped in the resulting blood clot. Blood bank work includes testing cells for the presence of antigens, and these particles may interfere with accurate results.

4.025 Which of the following tests in Blood Bank are sometimes done from a lavender-topped tube?
A. Type and crossmatch
B. Type and screen
C. Platelet count
D. Direct Coombs'

D. is the correct answer.

Sometimes a false-positive test result on a direct Coombs' test is obtained because of interference from blood calcium. EDTA anticoagulant (the anticoagulant of lavender tubes) prevents clotting by binding to calcium, rendering it unavailable to participate in the clotting process. Plasma from an EDTA tube therefore will be free of the interfering calcium.

4.026 Royal blue-topped tubes may contain the anticoagulant sodium heparin. How do they differ from green-stoppered tubes containing sodium heparin?
A. There is no difference, they can be used interchangeably
B. Royal blue-topped tubes never contain the anticoagulant sodium heparin
C. Royal blue-stoppered tubes have been acid washed to make them suitable for collection of certain trace elements, most notably lead
D. Royal blue-topped tubes containing sodium heparin utilize a special isomer of sodium

C. is the correct answer.

4.027 What blood protein can be found in plasma, but not in serum?
A. Hemoglobin
B. Fibrin
C. Fibrinogen
D. Albumin

C. is the correct answer.

Hemoglobin is a blood protein found in RBCs; its function is to carry oxygen.
Albumin is a protein that is found in serum and plasma.
Fibrinogen is a protein that is found in plasma, but when the blood clots, it changes into a stringy, ropey form called fibrin that is entangled in the blood clot.

4.028 What coagulation test is collected in an FDP tube?
A. PT
B. PTT
C. Fibrin degradation products
D. BT

C. is the correct answer.

Fibrin clots naturally break down after forming, creating fibrin degradation products. If FDP are present in greater than normal numbers, this may be an indication of disseminated intravascular coagulation (a condition characterized by many small blood clots throughout the vascular system).

4.029 What are the anticoagulants in an FDP tube?
A. Trypsin inhibitor and thrombin
B. Sodium citrate
C. EDTA
D. Heparin

A. is the correct answer.

Sodium citrate is the anticoagulant found in light blue-stoppered tubes used in most coagulation testing.
EDTA is the anticoagulant found in lavender-stoppered tubes used in most hematology testing.
Heparin in some form is the anticoagulant of green-stoppered tubes.

4.030 Which of the following are the common tests that are collected in a green-stoppered tube?
A. NH_3
B. LE prep
C. K
D. All of the above

D. is the correct answer.

When potassium levels are being tested, plasma preserved with heparin is actually preferred over serum, since potassium can be released from platelets during clotting.
NH_3 levels are collected in green-stoppered tubes, kept on ice, then separated and tested soon after collection.
Lead levels are collected in a royal blue-topped tube.

4.031 Which of the following tests are collected in a light blue (sodium citrate)-stoppered tube?
A. PT and PTT only
B. PT and Plt
C. TP and PT
D. PT, PTT, fibrinogen and TT

D. is the correct answer.

Plt stands for platelets. A platelet count can be ordered singly, but is often included in the hematology test, the CBC (complete blood count).
TP stands for total protein. This can be ordered singly, but is usually ordered as part of the general chemistry profile.

4.032 Blood has been collected from a patient and has been drawn into a vacutube with a lemon yellow stopper. What department is this blood sample going to be delivered to?
A. Blood Bank
B. Chemistry
C. Hematology
D. Microbiology

D. is the correct answer.

This blood sample will be taken to the Microbiology department of the laboratory, where it will have a culture and sensitivity performed on it to determine if there are any pathogens present in the patient's blood, and, if so, which antibiotics will effect a cure. In other words, this is an alternative method for collecting a blood culture. (Refer to question 4.058).

4.033 What is the anticoagulant in the lemon yellow-stoppered tube referred to in question 4.032?
A. Sodium polyanethole sulfonate (SPS)
B. Sodium citrate
C. Sodium fluoride
D. Sodium chloride

A. is the correct answer.

4.034 Which of the following tests may be contaminated by wearing latex gloves?
A. CBC
B. General chemistry profile
C. Electrolytes
D. Type and screen

B. is the correct answer.

It is possible to create falsely elevated calcium results with the powder residue from powdered latex gloves. When drawing a specimen for this test, it is best to wear powder-free gloves. Most general chemistry profiles include a calcium test.

4.035 Under which of the following circumstances are skin punctures indicated?
A. When patients have poor peripheral circulation for any reason
B. When patients have fragile veins. Examples of these patients are burn, oncology, pediatric and geriatric patients
C. When veins are tiny, as in newborns
D. All of the above

D. is the correct answer.

4.036 How deep should a pediatric lancet puncture?
A. Less than 1 mm
B. No more than 1 mm
C. Less than 2.5 mm
D. At least 2.5 mm

C. is the correct answer.

4.037 How deep should a standard lancet puncture?
A. Less than 5 mm
B. Up to 5 mm
C. Less than 1 mm
D. Less than 2.5 mm

B. is the correct answer.

4.038 The type of lancet that has a spring-activated puncture blade that provides a consistent puncture depth for capillary blood draws is called a(n):
A. Scalpel
B. Surgicutt
C. Autolet
D. Laser

C. is the correct answer.

The Surgicutt device also has a spring-activated cutting blade. This device is used to perform a specific coagulation test, the bleeding time test. Refer to questions 7.056–7.061 in Section 7 for more information on the bleeding time test.

4.039 What is the maximum lancet length recommended in newborn heel puncture?
A. Less than 1.0 mm
B. Less than 1.5 mm
C. Less than 2 mm
D. Less than 2.5 mm

D. is the correct answer.

4.040 A phlebotomist is called to the nursery to draw blood for a CBC and neobili test on a newborn. Which of the following supplies will s/he use to collect this blood?
A. An amber-tinted microcontainer for the neobili to protect it from light, and a lavender-topped microcontainer for the CBC
B. A plain red-topped microcontainer (untinted) with no additives for the neobili and a lavender-topped microcontainer for the CBC
C. An untinted microcontainer with a gel separator for the neobili and a lavender-topped microcontainer for the CBC
D. A pediatric red-topped tube and a pediatric EDTA-containing tube

A. is the correct answer.

4.041 Which of the following should be used for capillary blood gas collection?
A. Red-banded Natelson tubes
B. Green-banded Natelson tubes
C. Blue-banded Natelson tubes
D. Black-banded Natelson tubes

B. is the correct answer.

Red-banded heparinized Natelson tubes contain the anticoagulant ammonium heparin; green-banded Natelson tubes contain either lithium heparin or sodium heparin. Ammonium heparin may have a deleterious effect on one of the analytes of a blood gas determination, the measurement of hydrogen ion concentration (pH).

4.042 What is the additive in a lavender-topped microcontainer?
A. There is no additive
B. EDTA, either on beads or coating the sides of the microcontainer
C. Sodium citrate, either on beads or coating the sides of the microcontainer
D. Heparin

B. is the correct answer.

4.043 Which of the following will prevent air bubbles from being collected in capillary tubes for blood gases?
A. Holding the capillary tube horizontal to the puncture site
B. Filling the tube to capacity to eliminate an air space
C. Sealing both ends with sealing caps or clay
D. All of the above

D. is the correct answer.

4.044 When collecting blood for capillary blood gases, the collector should insert a metal filing into the capillary tube before filling it with blood. What is this metal filing called?
A. An insert
B. A flea
C. A keeper
D. A sharp

B. is the correct answer.

4.045 Referring to question 4.044, what is the purpose of the flea?
A. It is used to mix the blood
B. It reduces interference by attracting the ions in the blood
C. It has a tag on it that allows identification of the sample
D. It acts as a blood preservative

A. is the correct answer.

Before both capillary tube ends are sealed, a doughnut-shaped magnet is slipped over the tube. After the tube is sealed, the blood is mixed with the anticoagulant by running the magnet up and down the shaft of the tube several times. The metal flea inside the tube will travel the length of the tube, pulled by the magnet, thereby mixing the contents.

4.046 The system of blood collection that involves prediluting the blood sample at the time of collection is the:
A. Butterfly collection system
B. Syringe collection system
C. Unopette system
D. Vacutainer system

C. is the correct answer.

4.047   When the Unopette system is used to collect blood:
    A. The contents of a calibrated capillary tube are discharged into a prefilled resevoir to create a prediluted sample
    B. A plastic pipette is used to deliver a specific volume of blood into a diluent
    C. Diluent is dispensed into the blood sample
    D. Nothing special is done, the Unopette system refers to the part of the hematology instrument that performs the diluting function

A. is the correct answer.

4.048   What is the definition of a hematocrit?
    A. The percentage of whole blood that is cells
    B. The percentage of whole blood that is RBCs
    C. The percentage of whole blood that is fibrinogen
    D. The percentage of whole blood that is plasma

A. is the correct answer.

4.049   What is a 'spun crit'?
    A. A theoretically configured hematocrit, based on the numbers of cells counted
    B. A collection of the patient's blood in a small-bore capillary tube and centrifugation of the tube in a special hematocrit centrifuge to obtain a packed-cell volume
    C. A theoretically configured hematocrit based on the hemoglobin level
    D. A buffy coat

B. is the correct answer.

4.050   Spun hematocrits should be collected in a small-bore heparinized capillary tube. This tube:
    A. Has a green ring at one end
    B. Has a blue ring at one end
    C. Has a red ring at one end
    D. Is plain, it has no colored rings

C. is the correct answer.

4.051   Vacutainers that are smaller versions of standard-size vacutainers are known as:
    A. Microcontainers
    B. Macrocontainers
    C. Pediatric vacutainers
    D. Small-size vacutainers

C. is the correct answer.

4.052   The correctly filled EDTA microcollection tube (microcontainer) is filled:
    A. Not past the bottom fill line
    B. Above the top fill line
    C. At least to the top fill line
    D. At least to the bottom fill line and not past the top fill line

D. is the correct answer.

4.053   A microcontainer's maximum volume of fill is:
    A. Between 2 and 3 ml
    B. $600\,\mu l$
    C. About ½ ml
    D. Not more than $10\,\mu l$

B. and C. are correct answers.

$500\,\mu l$ equals ½ ml.

4.054   What are the disposable adapters called that fit over the needle holder, so that after venipuncture, the adapter is pushed forward over the needle holder until it completely encases the needle?
A. Pro-Ject 2000 needle holder
B. Saf-T Clik and B-D Safety Lok
C. Acci-Gard reusable blood collection holder
D. There is no such adapter or needle holder

B. is the correct answer.

4.055   This adapter fits over the needle and needle holder. It employs a needle-ejection lever that is used to separate the needle from the needle holder directly into a puncture-resistant biohazard waste container. It is called a:
A. Pro-Ject 2000 needle holder
B. Saf-T Clik and B-D Safety Lok
C. Acci-Gard reusable blood collection holder
D. There is no such adapter or needle holder

A. is the correct answer.

4.056   The contaminated needle is mechanically retracted into the needle holder where it is sealed up in a cylinder. The collector can then retrieve the cylinder and dispose of it properly. This adapter can be used more than once. It is called a:
A. Pro-Ject 2000 needle holder
B. Saf-T Clik and B-D Safety Lok
C. Acci-Gard reusable blood collection holder
D. There is no such adapter or needle holder

C. is the correct answer.

4.057   Which of the following pieces of equipment is not necessary for arterial blood gas collection?
A. A heparinized glass or plastic syringe
B. Ice water for transport
C. A 1.5-inch, 22-gauge needle
D. A tourniquet

D. is the correct answer.

4.058   Blood collected for blood cultures is drawn into:
A. A vacutainer with the anticoagulant sodium polyanethole sulfonate (SPS)
B. A lemon yellow-stoppered tube
C. Blood culture bottles containing a nutrient broth
D. A syringe

A., B., C. and D. are all correct.

A lemon yellow-stoppered vacutube contains sodium polyanethole sulfonate. After blood is drawn into this tube, it is transferred in a timely manner to blood culture bottles. Blood for blood cultures may also be collected directly into blood culture bottles. Finally, blood for blood cultures may be collected into a syringe first, as long as it is transferred immediately to blood culture bottles, before it clots.

4.059 Blood culture bottles come in sets of two because:
    A. The chances of obtaining bacteria-laden blood are greater with larger samples of blood
    B. One bottle is incubated aerobically, the other anaerobically
    C. They don't come in sets of two, one bottle is filled and incubated anaerobically for 2 days and then is vented to create an aerobic environment
    D. It is simply a manufacturing preference; the bottles may be used one at a time

B. is the correct answer.

Bibliography

ALBA's Medical Technology, Board Examination Review. Vol I. 9th edn. Anaheim, CA: Berkeley Scientific Publications, 1980

Garza D, Becan-McBride K. *Phlebotomy Handbook*. 3rd edn. Norwalk, CT: Appleton and Lange, 1993

Pendergraph G. *Handbook of Phlebotomy*. 3rd edn. Philadelphia, London: Lea and Febiger, 1992

Scientific Products General Catalog, Products or Diagnostics, Industry and Science. 1991–1992

Phelan S. *Phlebotomy Techniques. A Laboratory Workbook*. Chicago, IL: ASCP Press, 1993

Vacutainer Brand Evacuated Blood Collection System. Franklin Lakes, NJ: Beckton Dickinson, 1995

Simplate for in vitro diagnostic use. Durham, NC: Organon Teknika Corporation, 1992

NCCLS Specimen Collection. *Procedure for the Collection of Diagnostic Blood Specimens by Venipuncture*. NCCLS Document H3-A3, Vol. 11, No. 10, July 1991

SECTION 5:   COLLECTION PROCEDURES

Objectives

- To recognize the importance of correct patient and sample identification
- To identify pertinent label information
- To identify potential site for venipuncture, skin puncture
- To be able to list the steps in the venipuncture/skin puncture procedure
- To describe the effects of the tourniquet, heat, fist clenching
- To describe proper needle insertion, withdrawal
- To list criteria for sample rejection
- To explain common phlebotomy complications
- To discuss blood smear preparation
- To define basal state

Key facts

A. Basal state and departures from basal state
1. Diet (fasting)
2. Exercise
3. Age
4. Stress
5. Diurnal variation
6. Posture
7. Geographic location
8. Tourniquet application

B. Patient identification

C. Specimen labeling

D. Venipuncture sites (arm, foot, wrist, hand, ankle) and skin puncture sites (finger, heel)

E. Special circumstances
1. IV therapy
2. Central lines

F. Facilitating skin or venipuncture
1. Tourniquet
2. Heat
3. Palpating
4. Clenching fist
5. Gravity (dangling arm)

G. Decontamination of the venipuncture site
1. Cleansing agents
2. Procedure

H. Venipuncture
1. Evacuated tube system
   a. Supplies
   b. Procedure
   c. Tube exchange (order of draw)
   d. Amount of draw
   e. Withdrawal of needle
   f. Postvenipuncture care

    2.   Syringe system
- a.   Supplies
- b.   Procedure
- c.   Transferring specimen to evacuated tubes (order of fill)
- d.   Postvenipuncture care
- e.   Indications for use

    3.   Skin puncture
- a.   Supplies
- b.   Depth of puncture (adult vs. pediatric)
- c.   Heel punctures
- d.   Finger punctures
- e.   Complications (osteomyelitis, hemolysis, tissue fluid contamination)
- f.   Procedure
- g.   Order of draw

I.   Sample requirements
1. Chemistry
2. Hematology
3. Immunohematology (Blood Bank)
4. Serology
5. Microbiology
6. Coagulation
7. Therapeutic drug monitoring

J.   Complications
1. Syncope
2. Failure to obtain blood
3. Hematoma
4. Petechiae
5. Edema
6. Obesity
7. IVs
8. Sclerosed/occluded veins
9. Hemoconcentration
10. Hemolysis
11. Collapsed veins
12. Allergies
13. Thrombosis
14. False-positive/false-negative results with blood cultures

K.   Specimen rejection
1. Incorrectly labeled tubes
2. Unlabeled tubes
3. Hemolysis
4. Outdated tubes
5. Wrong collection tube
6. Blood collected at the wrong time
7. Insufficient sample
8. Interfering substances
9. Improper storage and/or transport

L.   Blood smears
1. Uses for blood smear
2. Criteria for a good-quality smear
3. Procedure for making smear
4. Problems with slide preparation

Questions and Answers

5.001   A person who has been fasting for 12 hours, is in a resting state, free from stress (including the stress of recent exercise), not pregnant, and not under the influence of alcohol, drugs or medications is said to be in:
    A. A state of diurnal variation
    B. A basal state
    C. A circadian rhythm
    D. A coma

B. is the correct answer.

Note: diurnal variations are normal variations in the concentrations of many of the substances in our blood at various times of the 24-hour day. It is traditional to assume that the chemical make-up of our blood in the early morning hours represents our basal state.

5.002   Which of the following describes a properly fasting patient?
    A. A patient who has refrained from all food and drink (except water) for at least 2 hours
    B. A patient who has refrained from all solid food for 8 hours
    C. A patient who has refrained from all food and drink (except water and black coffee) for 12 hours
    D. A patient who has refrained from all food and drink (except water) for 12 hours

D. is the correct answer.

Coffee (even when black) should not be consumed during a fast because it can mobilize cholesterol from the liver, falsely elevating cholesterol results.

5.003   Which of the following pre-venipuncture preparations is the most important?
    A. Wash hands and don gloves
    B. Consult the patient's requisitions
    C. Confirm the patient's identity
    D. Thoroughly cleanse the venipuncture site

C. is the correct answer.

Although all of the preparations listed are necessary, confirming the patient's identity is the most important task to perform prior to a venipuncture.

5.004   Which of the following is generally a fasting specimen? (A specimen to be collected when the patient is in a fasting state).
    A. An electrolyte panel
    B. A liver profile
    C. A cardiac profile
    D. A general chemistry profile

D. is the correct answer.

Cholesterol and glucose tests both require a fasting specimen. Cholesterol and glucose tests are included in most general chemistry profiles.

5.005   Which of the following is generally a fasting specimen (a specimen to be collected when the patient is in a fasting state)?
    A. Thyroid tests (T_3, T_4, TSH, FT_4, T_3U)
    B. Type and screen
    C. CBC
    D. Lipid profile

D. is the correct answer.

Lipid profiles include the following tests: Chol, Trig, HDL (high-density lipoprotein), LDL (low-density lipoprotein) and a Chol/LDL (ratio). These cholesterol tests require a fasting specimen.

5.006   Which of the following is generally a fasting specimen (a specimen to be collected when the patient is in a fasting state)?
A. NH_3
B. RBC folate
C. Rubella
D. Blood cultures

B. is the correct answer.

Note: this specimen is unusual in that it is generally considered to be a chemistry specimen but it is collected in an EDTA tube.

5.007   Which of the following specimens should be collected in a lavender-topped tube?
A. A CBC
B. An Hgb A_1C (glycosolated hemoglobin)
C. RBC folate
D. All of them

D. is the correct answer.

5.008   A phlebotomist prepares to draw the blood of a conscious and lucid patient. She notices that the patient is not wearing an identification wristband. How should she proceed?
A. She should check the name on the chart at the foot of the bed
B. She should ask the patient to state his or her full name
C. She could provide the patient with a name and ask the patient to confirm it
D. She should have the charge nurse identify the patient

B. is the correct answer.

The charge nurse could identify the patient, but if the patient is conscious and lucid, s/he may identify her/himself.

5.009   A phlebotomist preparing to draw the blood of a patient who does not appear to be alert, notices that there is no identifying wristband. How should the phlebotomist proceed?
A. He should ask family members who are present in the room to confirm the patient's ID
B. By providing the patient with a name, he can probably get the patient to affirm or negate it
C. He should have the charge nurse identify the patient
D. He should check the name on the chart at the foot of the bed

C. is the correct answer.

5.010   Whether computer-generated labels are used for labeling a blood specimen, or the specimen is labeled by hand, which of the following information need not be included?
A. Name of the patient
B. Identifying information such as a birth date or an identification number
C. Date and time of the draw
D. A., B. and C. are all vital information

D. is the correct answer.

5.011 Which of the following cannot be computer generated, and so must be added to a computer-generated label by hand?
A. The collector's initials
B. The patient's initials
C. The patient's social security number
D. Special instructions

A. is the correct answer.

5.012 Which vein of the forearm is the preferred vein for venipuncture?
A. The dorsal hand veins
B. The mediancubital
C. The cephalic
D. The basilic

B. is the correct answer.

The mediancubital is usually the first choice for venipuncture, followed by the cephalic and then the basilic. The mediancubital is the preferred vein because it is generally the best anchored by surrounding muscle. There are many variations in human vascular anatomy, so the phlebotomist should use the vein that s/he thinks will be the best choice.

5.013 Why should a phlebotomist always perform a venipuncture below an IV?
A. It is more comfortable for the patient
B. It is easier to obtain the blood from below an IV
C. So that the blood sample will not be contaminated with IV solution
D. It is traditionally done this way

C. is the correct answer.

5.014 If a phlebotomist must draw from above an IV site, how much blood should be drawn and discarded to avoid or minimize IV contamination?
A. The initial 1 ml of blood drawn
B. The initial 2–5 ml of blood drawn
C. The initial 5–10 cc of blood drawn
D. The initial 5–10 ml of blood drawn

C. and D. are the correct answers.

A cubic centimeter (cc) and a milliliter (ml) are the same amount, so C. and D. are the same answer.

5.015 What is the name of the venipuncture site when blood is obtained from the back of the hand?
A. The dorsal hand site
B. The ventral hand site
C. The metacarpal site
D. The digital site

A. is the correct answer.

5.016 The preferred site for drawing a blood sample is in the 'crook of the elbow'. This is known as the _____________ site.
A. Intercostal
B. Thoracic
C. Medial
D. Antecubital

D. is the correct answer.

5.017 When a blood sample must be obtained from a central line, which of the following is not the role of the phlebotomist?
A. To draw the blood carefully, maintaining strict sterile technique to avoid septicemia and discarding initial blood to avoid contamination
B. The phlebotomist should advise the person doing the collection of the volume needed for all tests
C. Upon receiving the sample from the collector, the phlebotomist should distribute the sample to the appropriate vacuum tubes
D. The phlebotomist should label the tubes correctly, and make note that the draw was a line draw

A. is the correct answer.

A central line is intravenous tubing that is inserted into a patient's vein for the purpose of administering fluids and medications, or for obtaining blood samples. Only authorized personnel may obtain blood from a central line; generally, this means nurses and physicians.

5.018 When a phlebotomist is making a second attempt to draw blood after an unsuccessful first attempt, which of the following techniques may help to ensure a successful venipuncture?
A. Applying heat to the venipuncture site
B. Striking or rapping the venipuncture site lightly
C. Instructing the patient not to 'hyperextend' their arm
D. All of the above are helpful

D. is the correct answer.

5.019 Patients may be instructed to 'clench and unclench their fist' several times after the tourniquet has been applied to help raise the vein. If this instruction is given, what precautions should be taken?
A. The phlebotomist should note the location of a suitable vein, loosen the tourniquet for a few minutes, then reapply and perform the venipuncture without allowing the patient to pump their fist
B. The phlebotomist should wait at least 1 minute after the vein has been raised before performing the venipuncture
C. The phlebotomist should perform the venipuncture as usual, but make a note on the label that the patient was instructed to pump his/her hand prior to the draw
D. No special precautions are necessary

A. is the correct answer.

This is because 'pumping the fist' after the tourniquet has been applied can alter some of the levels of some of the constituents in the blood, resulting in false values.

5.020 When the evacuated tube method for venipuncture is used, what is the correct order in which tubes should be filled?
A. Blood culture bottles, red-topped or SST tubes, light blue-topped tubes, lavender-topped tubes and finally any other anticoagulant-containing tube
B. Light blue-topped tubes, lavender-topped tubes, blood culture bottles, red-topped or SST tubes and finally any other anticoagulant-containing tube
C. Blood culture bottles, light blue-topped tubes, lavender-topped tubes, red-topped or SST tubes and finally any other anticoagulant-containing tube
D. None of the above

A. is the correct answer.

When utilizing the vacuum tube system, red-topped tubes are drawn before a tube for coagulation tests so that thromboplastin in the tissues will be deposited in the red-topped tube and will not contaminate the citrate tube.

5.021 Ideally, all tubes should be filled to within 10% of their labeled draw. For a tube containing an anticoagulant, a *minimum* fill of _________ is recommended.
A. 10%
B. 25%
C. 50%
D. 75%

C. is the correct answer.

5.022 In what order should vacutubes be filled from a syringe?
A. Blood culture bottles, light blue-topped tubes, lavender-topped tubes, any other anticoagulant-containing tube and finally red-topped or SST tubes
B. Light blue-topped tubes, lavender-topped tubes, blood culture bottles, red-topped or SST tubes and finally any other anticoagulant-containing tube
C. Blood culture bottles, light blue-topped tubes, lavender-topped tubes, red-topped or SST tubes and finally any other anticoagulant-containing tube
D. None of the above

A. is the correct answer.

In the case of a syringe draw, the blood is homogeneously mixed throughout the syringe and there is no point in trying to avoid including the thromboplastin in the citrate tube (see answer to question 5.020).
Because the blood was first drawn into a syringe, there has been a slight delay, and the clotting factors in the blood begin to activate immediately. For this reason, it is a good idea to empty the blood into the tube for coagulation tests as soon as possible. For the same reason, the tube that can tolerate a clot will be filled last.

5.023 Under what circumstances is a syringe used rather than a vacutube system?
A. When drawing a patient with low blood pressure or low blood volume
B. When drawing a dehydrated patient
C. When drawing older, oncology or burn patients
D. All of the above

D. is the correct answer.

Any time the collector feels that the patient's veins are going to be intolerant of the vacutube system, the syringe system may be a possible alternative.
Reasons for intolerance include A., B. and C.

5.024 Which of the following is not an acceptable area of the body for skin puncture?
   A. The heel, medial to an imaginary line drawn from great toe to heel, and areas that are lateral to an imaginary line drawn from pinkie toe to heel
   B. The heel, between imaginary lines drawn from the great toe to heel, and from the pinkie to the heel
   C. The distal, dorsal aspects of the fingers
   D. The ear lobe

B. is the correct answer.

Skin punctures must be performed to the outside of imaginary lines drawn from the great toe to the heel, and from the pinkie toe to the heel.

5.025 Why is it desirable to use a lancet to cut across the fingerprints rather than parallel with the fingerprints when performing a skin puncture?
   A. If the cut is made parallel with the fingerprints, the specimen is more likely to be contaminated
   B. If the cut is made parallel with the fingerprints, the blood will be likely to run down the channels of the prints, making it difficult to direct into a collection device
   C. The correct procedure is to make the cut parallel with the fingerprints
   D. It doesn't matter if the cut is made parallel to or across the fingerprints

B. is the correct answer.

5.026 When performing a skin puncture, the lancet should be held:
   A. Oblique to the fingerprints, at a 45° angle to the skin surface
   B. Oblique to the fingerprints, at a 15° angle to the skin surface
   C. Perpendicular to the fingerprints, at a 90° angle to the skin surface
   D. Perpendicular to the fingerprints, at a 45° angle

C. is the correct answer.

5.027 Why is it important to wipe away the first drop of blood that appears after a skin puncture is performed, before filling the microcontainers?
   A. The first drop of blood is often mixed with tissue fluid and might contaminate the sample
   B. The first drop of blood contains an abnormally high number of platelets
   C. The first drop of blood has a large number of clotting factors and will cause the blood to clot even if collected with anticoagulant
   D. It is not necessary to wipe away the first drop of blood

A. is the correct answer.

5.028   When obtaining blood by means of a skin puncture, the tests for which department are collected first?
A. Coagulation
B. Hematology
C. Chemistry
D. Blood Bank

B. is the correct answer.

Hematology specimens should be collected first because blood tends to clot from skin-puncture sites. Coagulation tests cannot be performed from blood collected by skin puncture. Chemistry and Blood Bank usually employ clotted blood, so these are collected after the Hematology specimens.

5.029   Which of the following may cause hemolysis of the specimen collected by skin puncture?
A. Not allowing the alcohol used in site preparation to dry completely
B. Squeezing the puncture site too hard, rather than 'milking' it moderately
C. Touching the tip of the collection scoop to the drop of blood
D. All of the above may cause hemolysis

A. and B. are the correct answers.

It is important to remember not to actually touch the collection device to the wound. A drop of blood should be allowed to form, and the scoop of the collection device should be touched to that.

5.030   What is the recommended tip length of a lancet to be used on neonates?
A. Less than 1.0 mm
B. 1.0–1.5 mm
C. 2.0–2.5 mm
D. Less than 2.5 mm

D. is the correct answer.

The lancet tip length used on neonates should be less than 2.5 mm. More recently, there has been concern that a puncture depth of 2.4 mm on a neonate is too deep. Some commercial neonate lancets are designed to puncture to a depth much less than 2.4 mm.

5.031   If the lancet used in a neonatal heel puncture cuts too deeply, what type of medical problem may result?
A. Calcaneous, an infection of the heel bone, may result
B. Osteomyelitis, an infection of the heel bone, may result
C. Septicemia may result
D. Toxemia may result

B. is the correct answer.

Calcaneous is the name of the large heel bone that may develop osteomyelitis if punctured. Septicemia is an infection of the blood, and toxemia is the presence of toxins in the blood.

5.032   A CBC and electrolytes were collected from a heavily bruised area. How might the results be affected?
A. The cell counts of the CBC and the potassium test of the electrolyte panel may be falsely elevated
B. The cell counts of the CBC and the potassium test of the electrolyte panel may be falsely lowered
C. The cell counts of the CBC may be falsely elevated and the potassium falsely lowered
D. The cell counts of the CBC may be falsely lowered and the potassium falsely increased

D. is the correct answer.

Blood drawn from a bruised area may be hemolysed. The CBC test counts the number of red blood cells in the blood. If the blood cells are lysed, or ruptured, this will falsely lower the number of red blood cells counted.
The electrolyte panel includes a test for the measurement of potassium in the blood. The level of potassium inside the red blood cells is much higher than the potassium in the plasma portion of blood. If the cells have ruptured and spilled their contents into the plasma, this can falsely elevate the potassium results.

5.033   What are some possible phlebotomist errors that may result in a hematoma (bruise)?
    A. A needle being inserted too deeply so that it goes completely through the vein
    B. Not inserting the needle deeply enough into the vein so that the opening of the needle is partially out of the vein
    C. Excessive 'probing' to find a missed vein
    D. All of the above

D. is the correct answer.

5.034   Which of the following is appropriate post-venipuncture care?
    A. Having the patient bend his or her elbow to apply constant pressure to the venipuncture site
    B. Application of a Band-Aid to supply adequate pressure to the venipuncture site
    C. Application of pressure to the venipuncture site while the patient holds his or her arm out straight
    D. It is not recommended to apply pressure to a venipuncture site, postvenipuncture

C. is the correct answer.

5.035   What is one of the first signs that a patient may be about to lose consciousness?
    A. The patient slumps forward
    B. The patient starts speaking incoherently
    C. The patient begins to perspire in the antecubital area
    D. The patient informs the phlebotomist that s/he is about to faint

C. is the correct answer.

Often the first sign that a patient is about to lose consciousness is the appearance of light perspiration in the crook of the elbow. If the patient complains of feeling faint, the draw should be stopped, and the patient should lower his/her head between the knees. An ammonia inhalant may be helpful to revive the patient. If the patient actually does faint, attempt to withdraw the needle and most importantly, prevent the patient from falling.

5.036   What is a hematoma?
    A. A blood clot in the soft tissue
    B. A blood clot in a blood vessel
    C. A collection of small hemorrhages, appearing as red dots in the affected area
    D. An *in vitro* blood clot

A. is the correct answer.

B. is a description of a thrombus. C. is a description of petechiae. D. is merely a blood clot that has formed in a test tube.

5.037   Which of the following may cause hemolysis?
    A. Use of a very-small-bore needle
    B. Too much back pressure (a concern in syringe draws)
    C. Inversion of tubes too vigorously
    D. All of the above

D. is the correct answer.

5.038   Excessive fluid build-up in the tissues is called:
    A. Sclerosis
    B. Eczema
    C. Edema
    D. Thrombosis

C. is the correct answer.

5.039   Why should edematous areas be avoided for venipuncture?
A. Blood may be difficult to obtain from an edematous area
B. Blood drawn from an edematous area may be contaminated with the tissue fluid
C. It is usually a painful venipuncture
D. People with edema should never have their blood drawn

A. and B. are the correct answers.

5.040   In what way can falsely lowered results be potentially harmful to the patient?
A. A patient's true results may be above normal, but if falsely lowered, may make the patient appear to be normal
B. Falsely lowered results may make the patient appear to have results that are below the acceptable range of normality
C. Generally speaking, falsely lowered results are not as serious as falsely elevated results
D. With state-of-the-art instrumentation, it is nearly impossible to obtain falsely lowered results

A. and B. are the correct answers.

5.041   While choosing a site for venipuncture, a phlebotomist notices that the patient's arms are covered with tiny red dots. What are these dots, and should they be of any concern to the phlebotomist?
A. They may be petechiae (tiny hemorrhages) and are of no concern to the phlebotomist
B. They may be petechiae and they should alert the phlebotomist to a potential bleeding problem
C. They are probably a rash and are of no concern to the phlebotomist
D. They are probably one of the viral diseases such as measles or chicken pox

B. is the correct answer.

When petechiae exist, the collector should be alerted to the fact that the patient may bleed abnormally. An alternative site should be chosen for venipuncture. Additionally, after the venipuncture is completed, longer pressure should be applied as part of postvenipuncture care.

5.042   Which of the following techniques probably will not be helpful in obtaining a blood specimen from a patient who is obese?
A. Do not allow the patient to hyperextend his/her arm when presenting it for phlebotomy
B. Obese patients are often easier to draw if they are not allowed to clench their hand prior to the stick
C. Use the syringe assembly; it is generally more effective on the obese patient
D. Apply the tourniquet more tightly

C. is the correct answer.

5.043   Veins that are obstructed are said to be
_______________; hardened veins are said to be
_______________:
A. Occluded, sclerosed
B. Sclerosed, occluded
C. Lipemic, icteric
D. Thrombosed, scarred

A. is the correct answer.

Lipemic refers to a high lipid or fat content in the serum, giving it an opaque, milky appearance. Icteric serum is the greenish hued serum sometimes seen in patients with liver disease. Thrombi are blood clots in the blood vessels. A thrombus may partially or fully occlude a vein. Veins often are sclerosed due to scarring.

5.044   Which of the following will not be helpful in dealing with a collapsed vein?
A. Repositioning the needle may alleviate the collapse
B. Removing the evacuated tube off the needle, and allowing the vein to refill with blood, then replacing the vacutube
C. Removing the tourniquet and allowing the blood flow to resume, and then tying off the tourniquet again
D. Tightening the tourniquet to build additional pressure

D. is the correct answer.

5.045   What should the collector do if there is a thrombus in the vein at a chosen venipuncture site?
A. Draw the blood anyway, taking great care not to disturb the thrombus
B. Choose an alternative site for venipuncture
C. Draw the blood from original site using the syringe system and a small-bore needle
D. Patients with thrombi should not be drawn from any site, unless done by a physician

B. is the correct answer.

5.046   When therapeutic drug levels are ordered, the appropriate way to collect them is to obtain a baseline _________ level, and a ________ level, or the level at which the medication is at its highest level in the patient.
A. Low; high
B. Valley; peak
C. Trough; peak
D. Minimum; maximum

C. is the correct answer.

5.047 In order to obtain the 'trough' level, the phlebotomist draws the patient's blood:
  A. Before the medication is administered
  B. Immediately after the medication has been administered
  C. At 08.00 hours
  D. At 24.00 hours (midnight)

A. is the correct answer.

In order to obtain the 'trough' level, the phlebotomist draws the patient's blood before the medication is administered. The phlebotomist then informs the nursing personnel that the trough level has been drawn. The medication is administered, and the phlebotomist returns at a predetermined time to obtain another blood sample. The timing of therapeutic drug monitoring is vitally important. The various medications given to patients have been analyzed to determine how long it should take for that particular medication to reach its highest concentration or 'peak' level in the blood, and this is when the second sample should be obtained. The phlebotomist should adhere to these guidelines in order to obtain an appropriate sample.

5.048 While loading a centrifuge, a technologist notices that one of the tubes is unlabeled. What is the appropriate course of action now?
  A. By process of elimination, it should be determined which patient the sample is from, and the tube can now be labeled
  B. By process of elimination, it should be determined which patient the sample is from, and the patient must be redrawn
  C. The entire unit that the patient is on will need to be redrawn
  D. By process of elimination, it should be determined which patient the sample is from, but if the results are normal they can safely be assigned to the patient

B. is the correct answer.

5.049 While drawing blood from a patient, a phlebotomist notices that the patient has a bottle of aspirin sitting on his nightstand. He asks the patient if he is taking aspirin, and the patient replies in the affirmative. Back in the lab, the phlebotomist makes note of this fact in the computer. Which of the following tests are likely to be affected by aspirin?
  A. Glucose
  B. CBC
  C. PT, PTT
  D. BUN

C. is the correct answer.

Aspirin changes the ability of blood to clot, so coagulation tests done on a patient who is taking aspirin may yield incorrect results.

5.050 Which of the following is not a reason for specimen rejection?
  A. Outdated tubes
  B. Unlabeled tubes
  C. Hemolysis of specimen
  D. Difficult draw

D. is the correct answer.

5.051   Which of the following is not a reason for specimen rejection?
   A. Incorrect collection tube
   B. Insufficient sample
   C. Interfering substances
   D. Improper storage and/or transit of the specimen

There are no correct answers.

These are all valid reasons for specimen rejection.

5.052   Blood for a CBC is initially drawn on a patient. Later, a glycosylated hemoglobin test is requested on this patient. Since the CBC and the hemoglobin A_1C (glycosylated HgB) are both done on EDTA anticoagulated blood, does the patient need to be drawn again?
   A. Yes, since the glycosylated hemoglobin requires a completely full EDTA tube
   B. Yes, since the glycosylated hemoglobin requires an unopened EDTA tube
   C. In all probability since the glycosylated hemoglobin needs to be collected on ice and the CBC probably wasn't collected this way
   D. No, the EDTA tube collected for the CBC will provide a good sample for the glycosylated hemoglobin

C. is the correct answer.

5.053   When anchoring a vein for venipuncture, the collector should:
   A. Anchor securely, with one finger above and one finger below the venipuncture site
   B. Anchor with one finger above the venipuncture site, pulling the skin taut
   C. Anchor with one finger below the venipuncture site
   D. It is not safe to anchor; most venipunctures can be performed without anchoring

C. is the correct answer.

Veins chosen for venipuncture are anchored with the phlebotomist's fingers to prevent their movement as the needle enters them. The vein chosen for venipuncture is anchored with one finger below the venipuncture site. Anchoring with two fingers, one above the venipuncture site and one below, is very dangerous. Theoretically, the phlebotomist's finger below the venipuncture site could be accidentally punctured but the chances of a needle puncturing a finger placed above the venipuncture site are greater.

5.054   Which laboratory department utilizes blood smears as part of their sample requirements?
   A. Microbiology
   B. Hematology
   C. Both Microbiology and Hematology
   D. All of the laboratory departments

C. is the correct answer.

The Microbiology department may Gram stain smears of blood to look for bacteria from blood cultures, but generally blood smears are made for the Hematology department. These smears are usually stained with Wright's stain, and various information is obtained by microscopic observation of the smears.

5.055 Briefly, a differential count that is done with a Wright-stained blood smear can be described as follows:
   A. It is a tally of the percentage (out of 100 WBCs counted) of different types of WBCs
   B. It is a tally of the different types of neutrophils noted in 100 WBCs counted
   C. It is a proportion of RBCs to WBCs
   D. It is a tally of the percentage (out of 100 RBCs counted) of different types of RBCs

A. is the correct answer.

5.056 In addition to a tally of the different types of WBCs, which of the following information may be obtained from a differential?
   A. Maturity of the WBCs present and the presence of any abnormal bodies or substances in the WBCs
   B. Morphology (shape) of RBCs present
   C. Approximate platelet morphology and count
   D. All of the above

D. is the correct answer.

5.057 A reticulocyte count reveals:
   A. Immature WBCs
   B. Immature RBCs
   C. Abnormal WBCs
   D. Abnormal platelets

B. is the correct answer.

EDTA-preserved blood is mixed with an equal amount of a special stain. After a short incubation time, a drop of this blood–stain mixture is used to make a smear on a microscope slide. The special stain reveals the presence of immature RBCs. Too many immature RBCs are not normal.

5.058 When making a blood smear, which preparations are considered to be good practice?
   A. Prepare immediately postdraw from blood containing no anticoagulant, or prepare from EDTA-anticoagulated blood
   B. Optimally, make within 1 hour of the draw and before the blood is refrigerated
   C. Blood sample should be well mixed before preparation of the smear
   D. All of the above

D. is the correct answer.

5.059 When referring to blood smears, what is a 'feathered' edge?
   A. It refers to the thin disbursement of blood cells at the end of a blood smear
   B. It is the portion of the smear that is viewed when doing a differential
   C. It is the outer edges on the sides of the blood smear
   D. It refers to an improperly prepared blood smear

A. and B. are the correct answers.

5.060   Why is it important not to allow the drop of blood that is used for a blood smear to sit on the slide for more than just a few moments before it is spread?
   A. The distribution of cells may be faulty
   B. The blood at the outer periphery of the blood drop may dry
   C. The interpretation of the differential may be inaccurate
   D. All of the above

D. is the correct answer.

If the drop of blood is allowed to sit for more than just a few moments, the distribution of cells may be faulty due to blood at the outer periphery of the blood drop drying, resulting in an inaccurate interpretation of the finished differential.

5.061   What causes some blood smears to appear to have 'waves' in the blood film, consisting of thick and thin distributions of blood cells?
   A. Depending on the hemoglobin content of the blood, this may be an inevitable result
   B. The fault lies with the manufacture of the microscope slide
   C. The pusher slide was not kept level and in constant contact with the smear slide
   D. High albumin levels in the blood cause this

C. is the correct answer.

5.062   How does a collector make a blood smear that has a feathered edge?
   A. The drop of blood used to make the smear should not be excessively large
   B. The pusher slide should be advanced all the way off the smear slide
   C. The pusher slide should be advanced rapidly
   D. All of the above

D. is the correct answer.

To obtain a feathered edge, the drop of blood should not be excessively large. Then the pusher slide should be advanced all the way off the smear slide; failure to do this will result in an abrupt edge rather than the desired 'feathered' edge. The pusher slide should be advanced fairly rapidly. A very slow push will result in the blood going off the end of the smear slide, again without a 'feathered' edge being formed.

Bibliography

NCCLS Specimen Collection. *Collection, Transport, and Preparation of Blood Specimens for Coagulation Testing and Performance of Coagulation Assays*. NCCLS Document H21-A, Vol. 6, No. 20, December 1986

NCCLS Specimen Collection. *Procedure for the Collection of Diagnostic Blood Specimens by Venipuncture*. NCCLS Document H3-A3, Vol. 11, No. 10, July 1991

NCCLS Specimen Collection. *Procedures for the Collection of Diagnostic Blood Specimens by Skin Puncture*. NCCLS Document H4-A3, Vol. 11, No. 11, July 1991

Garza D, Becan-McBride K. *Phlebotomy Handbook*. 3rd edn. Norwalk, CT: Appleton and Lange, 1993

Phelan, S. *Phlebotomy Techniques. A Laboratory Workbook*. Chicago, IL: ASCP Press, 1993

Pendergraph G. *Handbook of Phlebotomy*. 3rd edn. Philadelphia and London: Lea and Febiger, 1992

SECTION 6:   SPECIMEN PROCESSING (ORDERING, TRANSPORT, PROCESSING)

Objectives

- To explain the theory behind routine, ASAP, STAT and timed requests
- Knowledge of time constraints
- Knowledge of how to prioritize workload

Key facts

A.   Patient information
1.   Name
2.   Location
3.   Date and time specimen is to be collected
   a.   STAT
   b.   ASAP
   c.   Routine
   d.   Timed specimens
4.   Physician name, phone number
5.   Test requests
6.   Special instructions

B.   Routine and special procedures for transport
1.   Temperature
2.   Protection from light
3.   Aliquotting
4.   Pneumatic tube system of transport
5.   Dumbwaiters
6.   Hand carry by hospital personnel
7.   Postal service (shipping)
   a.   Shipping protocols
   b.   Labeling

Questions and Answers

6.001   When there is no particular priority assigned to the collecting and testing of a patient's blood, it is ordered as:
A. Basal
B. STAT
C. ASAP
D. Routine

D. is the correct answer.

6.002   Tests that are requested with STAT priority must get __________ priority:
A. Routine
B. Immediate
C. Timely, but not urgent
D. Timed

B. is the correct answer.

6.003   Test requests that include instructions that the blood be drawn at a particular time are known as:
A. Specific tests
B. Precise tests
C. Timed tests
D. All tests should be requested at specific times

C. is the correct answer.

6.004   Some tests by their nature have specific times attached to them. Generally, these tests will not include timing directions, it is up to the laboratory to understand the timing requirements, and to comply with them. Which of the following are examples of this type of test?
A. GTT
B. Therapeutic drug monitoring
C. GGT
D. CBC

A. and B. are the correct answers.

A GTT is a glucose tolerance test. First a fasting specimen is drawn from the patient. A glucose load is administered, and then blood specimens are drawn ½ hour, 1 hour, 2 hours etc. post-glucose load. Therapeutic drugs are drawn before the drug is administered and at various times after administration, depending on the drug. A GGT is a gamma-glutamyl transaminase. It is a liver function test and is not a timed test. A CBC is a complete blood count, also not timed test.

6.005   When a test is ordered ASAP, this means:
A. The test results are urgent
B. As soon as possible
C. The test should be performed in a timely but not urgent manner
D. The test is being performed postmortem

B. and C. are the correct answers.

6.006   When transporting specimens both in house, and when shipping between testing laboratories, which of the following should be adhered to?
A. The specimens should be kept on ice
B. The specimens should be protected from light
C. The specimens should be protected from excessive heat
D. The specimens should be kept upright

C. is the correct answer.

Specified specimens are kept on ice, but most specimens are kept at room temperature. Some specified specimens are protected from the light, but most can be exposed to light without harm. It usually does not matter if specimens are not kept upright during transit.

6.007 Which of the following specimens should be kept on ice after collection?
A. Glycosylated hemoglobin
B. NH_3
C. PTs and PTTs
D. All of the above

D. is the correct answer.

Since PTs and PTTs should have their tests performed within 2 hours of collection, some laboratories no longer require that they be on ice during this time.

6.008 Which of the following tests should be allowed to clot at 37 ℃?
A. Direct Coombs'
B. Cold agglutinins
C. Type and crossmatch
D. All blood bank tests

B. is the correct answer.

6.009 The lowest concentration of a therapeutic drug in the patient's blood that is usually drawn just before the medication is administered, is called the ________ level:
A. Peak
B. Bottom
C. Trough
D. Minimal

C. is the correct answer.

6.010 The ________ level is the highest concentration of the medication in the patient's blood.
A. Peak
B. Top
C. Trough
D. Maximal

A. is the correct answer.

6.011 Which of the following may affect the time it takes for a medication to reach its peak level in the blood?
A. The type of medication
B. The method of infusion (IM or IV)
C. The rate of infusion
D. All of the above

D. is the correct answer.

6.012 A Phlebotomy department receives the following orders on three different patients. A STAT glucose, an ASAP set of electrolytes, and a routine CBC. In what order should the tests be collected?
A. The glucose, the electrolytes and then the CBC
B. The electrolytes, the CBC and then the glucose
C. The phlebotomist should find out where the patients are, then s/he should start with the farthest one and quickly work his/her way back to the laboratory
D. It doesn't matter, these priorities apply to the testing technologist

A. is the correct answer.

STAT work gets first priority, followed by ASAP work. Routine work gets last priority.

6.013 Which of the following tests should be kept on ice following collection?
A. Cold agglutinins
B. CBC
C. Electrolytes
D. Renin activity

D. is the correct answer.

6.014   Which of the following tests should be protected from light after collection?
A. Any general chemistry panel
B. Electrolytes
C. Neobilirubin
D. Any coagulation test

C. is the correct answer.

6.015   Which of the following tests should be kept on ice following collection?
A. Serum hepatitis
B. Serum gastrin
C. Guaiac test
D. None of them

B. is the correct answer.

The guaiac test is a test for occult blood in (usually) stomach contents or a fecal sample.

6.016   What is the single *most* important procedure(s) for the phlebotomist to remember when collecting specimens for blood bank testing?
A. To draw the blood in a plain red-topped tube that doesn't have a gel barrier
B. To draw an EDTA tube in case extra testing such as direct Coombs' needs to be done
C. To correctly identify the patient and to correctly label all tubes
D. To draw all blood bank tests STAT

C. is the correct answer.

Although all of the choices are correct and should be followed, collectors should realize that because transfusion with inappropriate blood can be extremely dangerous for the patient, the most important procedures when collecting blood for any blood bank procedure are correct patient identification and correct tube labeling.

6.017   Which of the following information does not need to be verified when a testing laboratory receives a sample for testing?
A. The patient name and identification number on the sample should match the name and identification number on the test requisition form
B. The integrity of the specimen should have been maintained throughout its transport
C. The specimen type should be appropriate
D. All of the above are important and need to be verified

D. is the correct answer.

Additionally, there should be sufficient quantity of the specimen for the requested test(s) and patient history should be provided if appropriate.

6.018   What is the definition of an etiologic agent?
A. A viable micro-organism or its toxin that is capable of causing human disease
B. A pathogen
C. Any human material used for the purpose of diagnosis
D. A virus

A. and B. are the correct answers.

A diagnostic specimen is any human material, including but not limited to, blood and its components, excreta, secreta, tissue and tissue fluids, for the purpose of diagnosis. A virus can be an etiologic agent, but etiologic agents are not always viruses.

6.019   Which federal regulatory agencies' regulations must be met when shipping diagnostic specimens and etiologic specimens domestically?
A. The PHS and the DOT, respectively
B. OSHA
C. OSHA and the CDC, respectively
D. The United States Postal Service

A. is the correct answer.

The federal regulatory agency that has control over the domestic shipment of diagnostic specimens is the PHS (United States Public Health Service). The federal regulatory agencies that have control over the domestic shipment of etiologic specimens is the DOT (US Department of Transportation) and the PHS.

6.020   Which of the following choices is the correct procedure to follow when packaging a specimen for shipment to a reference laboratory?
   A. Primary container, absorbent material, outer shipping container, biohazardous label that includes the address and phone number of the CDC
   B. Primary container, durable secondary container, outer shipping container, biohazardous label that includes the address and phone number of the CDC
   C. Primary container, absorbent material, durable secondary container, outer shipping container, biohazardous label
   D. Primary container, absorbent material, durable secondary container, outer shipping container, biohazardous label that includes the address and phone number of the CDC

D. is the correct answer.

The primary container is the container that contains the specimen (such as a vacutube) and should be labeled with the patient's name and identification code. It is important to include absorbent material between the primary and secondary container sufficient to absorb the contents of the primary container in the event of leakage. The biohazardous label should include the address and the phone number of the CDC in the event of leakage.

6.021   How should frozen specimens be shipped in order to maintain their integrity during shipping?
   A. Frozen specimens are shipped in plastic vials
   B. Frozen specimens are maintained by shipping in an insulated package with dry ice
   C. If more than one test is ordered, frozen specimens should be aliquotted
   D. All of the above are necessary for shipping frozen specimens

D. is the correct answer.

Frozen specimens must maintain their integrity by shipping in plastic vials in an insulated package with dry ice. Be sure to submit individual frozen specimens for each test ordered since continual freezing and thawing can damage the integrity of the specimen.

6.022   What is the buffy coat?
   A. The layer of mostly WBCs and some RBCs that forms between RBCs and serum
   B. The layer of mostly WBCs and some RBCs that forms between RBCs and plasma
   C. A type of antibody
   D. A type of antigen

B. is the correct answer.

When anticoagulated blood is centrifuged, there is a grayish red layer of cellular components between the red blood cells on the bottom of the tube and the plasma layer on top. This cellular layer is comprised mostly of white blood cells and some red blood cells. This is the buffy coat, the layer that smears for lupus erthythematosis are made from.

6.023   Why is it important to draw a 'dummy' red-topped tube before drawing a citrate tube when collecting blood for coagulation tests?
   A. The 'dummy' red top is drawn in case the clinician has forgotten to order additional tests, so that the patient doesn't need to have another venipuncture
   B. The first substance that enters a needle that has been inserted through tissue for venipuncture is thromboplastin in the tissue. Since this will alter coagulation tests, it needs to be diverted into another tube
   C. It is not necessary to draw a 'dummy' red-topped tube before a citrate tube
   D. None of the above

B. is the correct answer.

6.024   After blood for coagulation testing has been transported to the laboratory, how should it be centrifuged?
A. At RCF of 1500 *g* for 5 minutes
B. At RCF of 1000 *g* for at least 10 minutes
C. At RCF of 5000 *g* for 30 minutes
D. It should not be centrifuged

B. is the correct answer.

6.025   Plasma that is to be used for coagulation testing should be removed from the RBCs and transferred to:
A. Glass test tubes
B. Fresh citrate tubes
C. Plastic or silicon-coated tubes
D. The plasma may sit on the RBCs until testing

C. is the correct answer.

The plasma can be stored, capped, at 0–8 °C for up to 4 hours. If it is not to be tested prior to this time frame, the plasma sample should be frozen until being tested.

6.026   Why is it advisable to separate serum or plasma needed for testing from the RBCs as soon as possible?
A. The results will be falsely elevated
B. The results will be falsely lowered
C. The results could be either falsely elevated or falsely lowered
D. It isn't necessary to separate the liquid portion of blood from the cellular portion

C. is the correct answer.

The liquid portion of the blood and the cells should not be in contact with each other for more than 2 hours. Many analytes tested exist in higher concentrations in RBCs than in serum or plasma. Diffusion out of the RBCs will falsely elevate analyte results.
Glucose concentrations will be lowered, because blood cells will continue to metabolize (break down) glucose even out of the body, causing glucose levels in the serum/plasma to lower.

6.027   What is the purpose of chilling specimens?
A. Chilling a specimen inhibits the metabolism of the blood cells
B. Chilling stabilizes thermolabile analytes
C. Chilling a specimen improves the quality of the clot formed
D. Chilling is detrimental in most cases

A. and B. are the correct answers.

Chilling a specimen inhibits the metabolism of the blood cells. Blood cells metabolize or break down the glucose in blood.
Chilling also stabilizes thermolabile analytes. Thermolabile refers to the tendency for certain substances to decompose, dependent upon temperature. Analytes that are thermolabile at room temperature may be stabilized at chilled temperatures.

6.028   A program or the methods used that will assure accuracy in any business is called:
A. Quality assurance
B. Quality control
C. Precision
D. Accuracy

A. is the correct answer.

The term 'quality assurance' implies a program or the methods used that will assure accuracy in any business. In the case of clinical medicine, the business is patient care.
The term 'quality control' implies the daily operational procedures followed by the care-giving institution in order to implement the quality assurance program.

Bibliography

NCCLS Specimen Collection. *Procedures for the Domestic Handling and Transport of Diagnostic Specimens and Etiologic Agents*. 2nd edn. NCCLS Document H5-A2, Vol. 5, No. 1, January 1985

NCCLS Specimen Collection. *Collection, Transport, and Preparation of Blood Specimens for Coagulation Testing and Performance of Coagulation Assays*. NCCLS Document H21-A, Vol. 6, No. 20, December 1986

NCCLS Specimen Collection. *Procedure for the Collection of Diagnostic Blood Specimens by Venipuncture*. NCCLS Document H3-A3, Vol. 11, No. 10, July 1991

NCCLS Specimen Collection. *Procedures for the Handling and Processing of Blood Specimens*. NCCLS Document H18-A, Vol. 10, No. 12, June 1984

American Association of Blood Banks Technical Manual. Philadelphia, Toronto: J.B. Lippincott Company, 1981

SECTION 7: SPECIAL COLLECTIONS AND SPECIAL HANDLING

Objectives

- To be able to define the steps necessary for the various types of tolerance testing
- To be able to define the steps necessary for the various types of urine collection
- To be able to recognize what kind of tests require special patient preparation
- To be able to recognize which tests require special handling
- To be able to correctly prep a patient and draw a blood culture
- To be able to correctly prep a patient and draw for legal and non-legal blood alcohols
- To be knowledgeable about the steps involved in an arterial blood gas draw

Key facts

A.   Bedside testing

B.   Tolerance testing
    1.   1-hour post-prandial glucose
    2.   3-, 4- and 5-hour glucose tolerance test
    3.   2-hour post-prandial test
    4.   Epinephrine tolerance test
    5.   D-Xylose tolerance test
    6.   Lactose tolerance test

C.   Urine specimen collection
    1.   Random specimen
        a.   Midstream
        b.   Clean catch
    2.   24-hour collection
    3.   Urine collection for culture
    4.   Urine collection for drug testing; NIDA sample collection

D.   Other body fluids
    1.   CSF
    2.   Gastric secretions
    3.   Synovial fluid
    4.   Pleural fluid
    5.   Pericardial fluid
    6.   Peritoneal fluid
    7.   Seminal fluid
    8.   Amniotic fluid

E.   Specimens greatly affected by hemolysis

F.   Specimens that must be transported on ice

G.   Specimens that must be protected from light

H.   Specimens that must be collected from a fasting patient

I.   Blood alcohols
    1.   Legal
    2.   Non-legal

J.   Blood cultures

K.   Arterial blood gases (Allen test)

L.   Therapeutic drug monitoring

M.   Throat culture

N.   Skin tests

O.   Sweat test

P.   Cold agglutinins

Q.   Renin activity test

R.   Hemoglobin A_1C test

S.   PKU testing

T.   Bleeding time test

Questions and Answers

7.001 What is a 'control'?
   A. A manufactured substance that resembles blood; it contains a known amount of analyte and is used to test an instrument's performance
   B. A manufactured substance that resembles blood; it is used to establish a reference point
   C. A guard on an instrument to ensure that it samples precisely
   D. A set of operating instructions designed to produce reliable results

A. is the correct answer.

Controls are treated identically to a patient sample. The control is introduced to the analyzing instrument following the same procedures that are recommended for patient testing. The instrument must be able to obtain a result that is within a close range of the known value of the control. The acceptable range of accuracy will be provided by the manufacturer of the control. Usually at least two controls are run on a daily basis, a low and a high control. It should be remembered that patient samples that are tested without a control being run are useless.

7.002 What is a 'calibrator'?
   A. A manufactured substance that resembles blood; it contains a known amount of analyte and is used to test an instrument's performance
   B. A manufactured substance that resembles blood; it is used to establish a reference point
   C. A guard on an instrument to ensure that it samples precisely
   D. Diluent

B. is the correct answer.

At least once a month, a calibration should be performed. A calibrator is a manufactured substance that contains a known amount of glucose. The analyzing instrument is set so that it is 'told' that the calibrator has, for example, 100 mg of glucose. The instrument will then store this information and compare all future samples, whether they be controls or patient samples, to the calibrator result in order to obtain a test result.

7.003 What is the first step of the GTT (glucose tolerance test) procedure?
   A. Obtain a fasting urine sample
   B. Obtain a fasting blood sample
   C. Do a fingerstick and test the blood with a glucose test strip
   D. Have the patient eat a high carbohydrate diet for 3 days prior to the test

D. is the correct answer.

The purpose of a glucose tolerance test is to determine how efficiently a patient is able to release insulin and move a known amount of glucose from the bloodstream to the tissue cells where the glucose can be oxidized for energy. Patient preparation involves having patient load carbohydrates for 3 days prior to the test. The patient should eat meals that include 150 g of glucose a day; some information as to how this can be done should be provided to the patient. Additionally, a 12-hour fast prior to the GTT is required.

7.004   Which of the following shows the correct order of operations when performing a GTT? (Assume the patient has loaded carbohydrates for 3 days prior to the test and has fasted for 12 hours.)
A.   Fingerstick glucose, fasting urine and blood samples obtained, glucose load given, blood samples obtained at 30 minutes, 1 hour, 2 hours and 3 hours post-glucose load
B.   Fingerstick glucose, fasting urine and blood samples obtained, glucose load given, blood and urine samples obtained at 30 minutes, 1 hour, 2 hours and 3 hours post-glucose load
C.   Fingerstick glucose, fasting urine and blood samples obtained, glucose load given, blood and urine samples obtained at 1 hour, 2 hours and 3 hours post-glucose load
D.   Fasting urine and blood samples obtained, glucose load given, blood and urine samples obtained at 30 minutes, 1 hour, 2 hours and 3 hours post-glucose load

B. is the correct answer.

After a 12-hour fast, the patient is tested to determine that his/her fasting glucose level is less than 150 mg/dl. If the test is to proceed, the patient is asked to give a urine sample and a blood sample. These are the fasting levels, and constitute the patient's baseline results.
Next, the known amount of glucose is administered to the patient. It comes in the form of a flavored drink. Some testing sites administer 100 g of glucose to all adult patients, and some sites administer the amount of glucose according to patient weight. The patient should make every attempt to drink the glucose solution within 5 minutes. Thirty minutes, 1 hour, 2 hours, 3 hours (and 4 and 5 hours if applicable) after the patient has finished ingesting the glucose, he/she gives a blood sample and a urine sample which will be tested for glucose levels, and for glucose and the presence of ketones, respectively. The results of the patient are compared to the results of normal glucose disposal.

7.005   What is the purpose of testing a fasting patient's glucose level with a fingerstick test prior to a GTT?
A.   It establishes the need to have a GTT performed
B.   It establishes whether or not the patient is truly fasting
C.   It ensures that the patient can tolerate a GTT
D.   It is not necessary to begin a GTT with a fingerstick glucose, this information will be obtained with the fasting blood sample

C. is the correct answer.

Since the patient will be given a glucose load, his/her fasting glucose level must be sufficinetly low so that the load will not increase his/her blood glucose up to dangerous levels. Generally, a GTT cannot proceed unless the patient's fasting glucose is at or below 150 mg/dl.

7.006   If a patient is lactase deficient, during an LTT (lactose tolerance test), s/he will exhibit a glucose curve that:
A.   Is much higher than his/her GTT glucose curve
B.   Is only slightly higher than his/her GTT glucose curve
C.   Is much lower than his/her GTT glucose curve
D.   Has no relation to his/her GTT glucose curve

B. is the correct answer.

The lactose tolerance test is used to evaluate a lactase deficiency. Lactase is a digestive enzyme that hydrolyzes lactose (milk sugar) into its constituent sugars, glucose and galactose.
On the day previous to the LTT, a 3-hour GTT must be performed to establish the patient's own normal glucose curve. On the following day, the LTT is performed in the same manner as the GTT. The same amount of lactose is administered to the patient as glucose was previously administered.
Blood samples are collected at the same intervals as in the GTT, and tested for glucose (one of the constituents of lactose, if lactose is being hydrolyzed normally).
The normal patient will exhibit a glucose curve after ingestion of lactose that will be similar to his/her glucose curve from the GTT. The lactase-deficient patient will only show a very slight increase in blood glucose.

7.007   Which tolerance test is used to screen pregnant patients for gestational diabetes?
A. The 3-hour GTT
B. The 5-hour GTT
C. The 1-hour PPG (post-prandial glucose) test
D. The 2-hour PPG test

C. is the correct answer.

To begin the test, the patient is asked to drink a standard dose of glucose (50 g) in a flavored beverage. The patient must start and finish the drink within 5 minutes.
When the patient has finished the glucose solution, the time is noted and a single blood sample for glucose is obtained after 1 hour. Abnormal glucose results may mean that a diabetic problem exists, and the patient may be evaluated further.

7.008   Which test is sometimes ordered prior to a full GTT, to eliminate the need for a GTT if the results are normal?
A. The 3-hour GTT
B. A FBS
C. The 1-hour PPG (post-prandial glucose) test
D. The 2-hour PPG test

D. is the correct answer.

Prandial is another name for meal. This test is used as a screen for diabetes. Because this test is so much less traumatic for the patient than a GTT, doctors will often order it first, and if the results are abnormal, then order the full GTT. For this test, the patient is instructed to eat a breakfast with approximately 100 g of glucose in it. Instructions advising the patient about the kind of menu that will include about 100 g of glucose are provided. Two hours after the meal, a blood sample is drawn for glucose determination. The normal 2-hour blood glucose level should be ≤120 mg/dl.

7.009   When collecting urine for a 24-hour creatinine clearance test, the patient should:
A. Collect the first morning void and all subsequent voids for the next 24 hours
B. Discard the first morning void, then note the time of the next void and collect it and collect subsequent voids for the next 24 hours
C. Discard the first morning void, but consider the time of that first void to be the beginning of the test, and collect subsequent voids for the next 24 hours
D. Simply start the 24-hour collection several hours after rising, and collect all voids during a 24-hour time frame

C. is the correct answer.

When collecting urine for a 24-hour collection, the first morning void at the beginning of the test should be discarded. Although this first void is discarded, the time that this is done should mark the beginning of the test. For example, if the patient voids for the first time at 07.00 hours, this should be discarded, but 07.00 should be written on the 24-hour collection container as the beginning of the 24-hour collection period. All urine voided during the next 24 hours should be collected. At 07.00 hours the following day, the patient should attempt to void one last time, and this should be added to the collection. If the patient is unable to void at this time, the collection is ended anyway.

7.010 Why is it important for the person receiving the 24-hour specimen at its completion to note the total volume of the specimen?
A. In case any of the sample is lost
B. It's not necessary to note the total volume
C. To ensure that there is sufficient sample
D. The results of analysis done on urine from a 24-hour collection are configured results, and the total volume must be calculated into the configuration

D. is the correct answer.

7.011 Patients collecting for a 24-hour collection should void into an alternative collection device first and then transfer the contents to the 24-hour collection container. What is the purpose of this?
A. To keep the sample uncontaminated
B. For ease of collection
C. To protect the patient from harmful substances in the 24-hour collection container
D. It's not necessary to do this

C. is the correct answer.

Many tests done with 24-hour urine collections involve the use of preservatives. Many of these preservatives are highly corrosive (HCl is a common preservative). If the patient voids directly into the collection container, there may be a splash effect and the patient could be injured.

7.012 When collecting samples that may involve civil or criminal law, very precise methods of collection, labeling and transport must be followed. These precise procedures are known as:
A. The 'Chain of Custody' of the sample
B. The 'Patients' Bill of Rights'
C. The 'Right to Know'
D. JCAHO's '10-Step Process'

A. is the correct answer.

These procedures involve accurate identification of the patient, the signatures of the employee(s) involved in the collection to verify the accurate labeling and safe transport of the specimen, and verification of the date, time and location of the sample collection are also included. The signature of the patient verifying that his/her sample is the one collected and labeled is required, and signatures of witnesses able to confirm that all the above statutes have been met are desirable. Personnel receiving the sample at the testing laboratory should verify that the specimen was received in an appropriate condition. A sample received in an appropriate condition means that the seals used to close the specimen container and its transport bag remain intact until the testing laboratory personnel break them. Any transfers involved in transport of the specimen should be documented.

7.013 The 'Chain of Custody' procedures with regard to urine collection must conform to _________________ requirements concerning collection, processing and transport of urine samples:
A. The Hippocratic Oath
B. NIDA (National Institute of Drug Abuse)
C. OSHA's Exposure Control Plan
D. The Clinical Laboratory Improvement Act

B. is the correct answer.

When collecting samples that may involve civil or criminal law, very precise methods of collection, labeling and transport must be followed. These precise procedures are known as the chain of custody of the sample. These procedures involve accurate identification of the patient, the signatures of the employee(s) involved in the collection to verify the accurate labeling and safe transport of the specimen, and verification of the date, time and location of the sample collection are also included. The signature of the patient verifying that his/her sample is the one collected and labeled is required, and signatures of witnesses able to confirm that all the above statutes have been met are desirable.
Personnel receiving the sample at the testing laboratory should verify that the specimen was received in an appropriate condition. A sample received in an appropriate condition means that the seals used to close the specimen container and its transport bag remain intact until the testing laboratory personnel break them.
Any transfers involved in transport of the specimen should be documented.

7.014 What kind of urine sample should a patient be asked to collect for a culture and sensitivity on a urine sample?
A. A random sample
B. A clean catch sample
C. A 24-hour sample
D. A catheterized sample

B. is the correct answer.

The patient should be instructed to obtain a clean catch specimen. It is important that debris and normal bacteria from the outside of the genitals be wiped away so that they will not contaminate the specimen. Women should separate the skin folds around the urinary tract opening, and cleanse this area well with the provided wipes. Continuing to hold the skin folds apart, she should begin to void, voiding at least half her urine before attempting to catch any. Without stopping the flow, the container should be placed into the stream to catch a portion of the urine. The collecting container should not be allowed to come into contact with the genital area. When a sufficient sample has been collected, she should continue to void into the toilet.

7.015   What is the difference between the routine urinalysis test and the urine test for culture and sensitivity?

A. The routine urinalysis investigates a urine specimen for various chemical and physical properties, and a urine culture and sensitivity examines urine for the presence of pathogens

B. The routine urinalysis investigates a urine specimen for the presence of pathogens, and the culture and sensitivity investigates a urine specimen for various chemical and physical properties

C. The routine urinalysis and a urine for culture and sensitivity are two names for the same test

D. The routine urinalysis test determines alcohol content of the urine and the urine for culture and sensitivity is a complete drug screen

A. is the correct answer.

A routine urinalysis test is a panel of tests that investigate a urine specimen for the presence of protein, glucose, ketones, urobilinogen, bilirubin, WBCs, nitrites and specific gravity. The urine sample that is tested for culture and sensitivity is examined for the presence of pathogenic bacteria. If a pathogen is found, a battery of antibiotics is tested against the organism to determine which ones will be capable of combating the infection.

7.016   Urine samples that are collected with no regard for time are called:

A. Routine samples
B. Random samples
C. Foley samples
D. Catheter samples

B. is the correct answer.

7.017   Clear fluid that surrounds the spinal cord and which is obtained by spinal tap is called:

A. Gastric secretions
B. Pleural fluid
C. Synovial fluid
D. Cerebral spinal fluid

D. is the correct answer.

7.018   Contents of the stomach, obtained via gastric intubation, are known as:

A. Gastric secretions
B. Pleural fluid
C. Synovial fluid
D. Cerebral spinal fluid

A. is the correct answer.

7.019   The fluid that surrounds the joints and is aspirated with a special needle is called:

A. Gastric secretions
B. Pleural fluid
C. Synovial fluid
D. Cerebral spinal fluid

C. is the correct answer.

7.020   Fluid from the lung cavity that is aspirated with a special needle is called:

A. Pericardial fluid
B. Pleural fluid
C. Peritoneal fluid
D. Amniotic fluid

B. is the correct answer.

7.021   Fluid from the abdominal cavity is called:
A. Pericardial fluid
B. Pleural fluid
C. Peritoneal fluid
D. Amniotic fluid

C. is the correct answer.

7.022   The fluid that surrounds the fetus in the uterus and should be protected from light is called:
A. Pericardial fluid
B. Pleural fluid
C. Peritoneal fluid
D. Amniotic fluid

D. is the correct answer.

7.023   Semen collected from males, usually for fertility studies, is known as:
A. Amniotic fluid
B. Peritoneal fluid
C. Seminal fluid
D. Synovial fluid

C. is the correct answer.

7.024   Which of the following tests can be greatly affected by hemolysis of the sample?
A. K (potassium)
B. Glucose
C. Type and crossmatch
D. Cold agglutinins

A., B., C. and D. are all correct.

Potassium levels inside the RBCs are much higher than K levels of the plasma. Hemolysis will increase serum or plasma levels.
Cells continuously use glucose for their metabolic processes. This will lower the glucose concentration in the specimen. A hemolyzed specimen will show the same effects as a sample in which serum has been allowed to remain on the cells; the glucose level will be falsely lowered.
The type and crossmatch tests donor and patient blood to ascertain which units of donated blood are compatible with a patient. Hemolyzed blood may obscure the true results.

7.025   Which of the following tests may be greatly affected by hemolysis?
A. Acid phosphatase
B. CBCs
C. Prostatic specific antigen
D. LDH

A., B. and D. are the correct answers.

Acid phosphatase is used to help detect cancer of the prostate, although a more current test is the PSA, the prostatic specific antigen. There is a prostatic and non-prostatic source; the non-prostatic source is in the RBCs. The CBC is the most commonly performed test in the Hematology department. An actual count of the RBCs is done as part of this test, so you don't want to 'lose' some of them to hemolysis.
LDH is an enzyme in tissue cells. When tissue cells become damaged, LDH is released into the blood. The presence of LDH can provide diagnostic information about disease; for example it is elevated after a heart attack. It is part of the cardiac profile and also of any basic chemistry profile. LDH is much higher in RBCs, so you don't want any to leak out into the serum and falsely elevate results.

7.026   Which of the following should be redrawn if the sample is hemolyzed?
A. RBC folate
B. Bilirubin
C. Cold agglutinins
D. CPK

B. and C. are the correct answers.

A liver function test, bilirubin is derived from hemoglobin, a protein found in RBCs. When doing a cold agglutinin test, either a true cold agglutination or hemolysis will give a positive result.

7.027   Which of the following should be collected on ice?
A. CBCs
B. Liver profiles
C. Renin activity
D. Electrolytes

C. is the correct answer.

This is helpful in diagnosing hypertension and should be collected under the following conditions:
a. The patient should maintain a normal salt intake for 3 days;
b. Diuretics and estrogen (oral contraceptives) should be discontinued for 2 weeks prior to the test;
c. Antihypertensive drugs should be discontinued several days before the test;
d. Either a standing or a recumbent order will be dictated by the ordering clinician;
e. Standing samples should be collected after the patient has been upright for 1 hour;
f. Recumbent samples should be collected after the patient has been recumbent for at least 30–45 minutes, preferably overnight;
g. The blood should be drawn into an EDTA-preserved (lavender-topped) tube that has been in an ice cup before drawing until it is thoroughly chilled. Draw blood into the cold tube and put back on ice.

7.028   Which of the following is the test that ought to be drawn on ice and from a fasting patient?
A. Serum folate
B. Serum folic acid
C. Serum gastrin
D. Gastric lavage

C. is the correct answer.

It should be noted that a serum folate and a serum folic acid are two names for the same test.

7.029   Which of the following is true of a legal blood alcohol test?
A. It is permissible to use an alcohol wipe to prep the venipuncture site
B. Legal blood alcohols are done for the protection of the patient
C. The patient cannot refuse a legal blood alcohol
D. The legal blood alcohol test actually consists of a panel of tests that constitute a complete drug screen

C. is the correct answer.

Legal blood alcohols are often collected to provide legal evidence concerning the suspect's level of blood alcohol. Specific procedures must be followed so that the evidence meets all the legal requirements. Procedures may vary between police departments, but these four procedures should always be followed:
a. Be certain of the identity of the patient;
b. Alcohol wipes should not be used to prepare the venipuncture site; instead, prepare the site with an iodine swab;
c. Note the time and date of the draw;
d. Be sure there is an officer present during the entire procedure, including the identification, the procedure and the labeling, who can sign as a witness.

7.030   In what way does a non-legal blood alcohol differ from a legal blood alcohol?
A. The testing procedures for a non-legal blood alcohol are not as thorough as for a legal blood alcohol
B. The legal blood alcohol is always performed at a police station, never in the hospital
C. The non-legal blood alcohol is performed for the safety of the patient
D. The patient may not refuse to have a non-legal blood alcohol done

C. is the correct answer.

Clinicians often order an alcohol to be drawn because they want to order medication for the patient and it is vitally important to know if the patient is under the influence of alcohol, which may contraindicate some medications. This is not a legal procedure, the patient may refuse. Care must be taken not to contaminate the venipuncture site with alcohol.

7.031   When drawing blood for blood cultures:
A. The aerobic bottle should be inoculated first
B. The anaerobic bottle should be inoculated first
C. The venipuncture site should be prepped twice with alcohol pads
D. The blood is always collected into a syringe

B. is the correct answer.

The anaerobic bottle should be inoculated first. The blood culture bottles contain a vacuum, and when a syringe or vacuum tube is discharged into them, the needle of the assembly will suck air as the needle is removed from the bottle. This means that the remaining contents of the discharging assembly will be aerated, or mixed with oxygen. At this point, the phlebotomist no longer has a sample that can be subjected to anaerobic conditions. If both blood culture bottles contain the same medium, this won't be a problem, since the first bottle inoculated can simply become the anaerobic bottle. In some institutions, the mediums of the anaerobic and the aerobic bottles differ, and, in this case, the phlebotomist must take care to inoculate the anaerobic bottle first.

7.032   Which of the following precautions should be taken when prepping a venipuncture site for blood cultures?
A. Iodine rather than alcohol should be used as a cleansing agent
B. The cleansing agent should be applied to the venipuncture site in concentric circles
C. The tops of the blood culture bottles should be cleansed before they are inoculated
D. All of the above

D. is the correct answer.

An iodine scrub should be employed to cleanse the venipuncture area. The iodine scrub contains iodine for antisepsis, and a lathering agent to help reduce the amount of bacteria on the skin. Instant antisepsis does not occur, so the iodine scrub should be employed for a minimum of 2 minutes. Next, an alcohol swab/prep should be used to remove excess lather from the venipuncture site. The venipuncture area is then prepped with a povidone iodine swab. The phlebotomist should start at the actual intended venipuncture site, and move outwards in concentric circles. If there are any remaining bacteria, this will serve to push them away from the venipuncture site. The area must be allowed to dry thoroughly. While the site is drying, the phlebotomist may prepare the tops of the blood culture bottles by cleansing the tops of the bottles with an iodine scrub. The iodine lather should be removed with alcohol prep pads.

7.033 What is generally considered to be the minimally acceptable sample size for a blood culture?
A. 5–10 cc total
B. 5–10 cc per bottle
C. 50 cc total
D. 300–350 ml total

B. is the correct answer.

Blood that is collected for blood cultures is placed in nutrient broth so that bacteria, if present, will be able to live and grow. It is generally considered that a nutrient broth of 10 times the volume of the inoculum is desirable. 5–10 cc of blood is considered to be a minimum amount of inoculum necessary for good recovery of organisms. Some bacteria are aerobic and prefer an environment with oxygen; some bacteria are anaerobic and prefer an environment lacking oxygen. For this reason, two nutrient broth bottles are inoculated when blood cultures are collected. One bottle is shunted to provide oxygen and the other is not, so as to provide an anaerobic environment. 5–10 cc of blood should be collected for *each* bottle.

7.034 Supposing a phlebotomist drawing blood for blood cultures is only able to obtain about 6 cc of blood. What should s/he do?
A. Divide the blood into the two blood culture bottles, one aerobic and the other anaerobic
B. S/he should divide the blood obtained into two pediatric blood culture bottles, one aerobic and one anaerobic
C. The blood should all be emptied into an aerobic bottle
D. The blood should all be emptied into an anaerobic bottle

C. is the correct answer.

Since a bacteremia is more likely to be caused by an aerobe rather than an anaerobe, it is better policy to go with the law of averages and inoculate the aerobic bottle.

7.035 Blood cultures are usually either drawn ×2 or ×3 at timed intervals or ×2 at the same time but at different locations on the body. What is the reason for this?
A. There are usually several infection sites that are making the patient ill
B. There is a greater likelihood of obtaining a blood specimen containing the pathogen
C. Blood cultures include sensitivities, and extra blood is needed for this
D. This isn't the way blood cultures are usually drawn

B. is the correct answer.

Blood cultures are usually either drawn ×2 or ×3 at timed intervals or ×2 at the same time but at different locations. Bacteria are not homogeneously distributed throughout the blood. Bacteria travel in boluses, and by collecting at different locations or at different times, you increase the chance of catching a bolus.
When a patient is ill with septicemia, his fever will spike when the bacteria travel through internal organs. After 15–30 minutes, the bacteria pass through the peripheral circulation, and this is when the BCs should be collected. BCs from two different sites at the same time are sometimes ordered. These are often referred to as 2nd-site blood cultures.

7.036 Give some reasons for false negatives in blood culture results due to poor phlebotomy technique.
A. Filling the aerobic bottle first
B. Failure to allow the venipuncture site or the iodine-cleansed bottles to dry
C. Too little volume drawn
D. All of the above

D. is the correct answer.

7.037 Give some reasons for false positives in blood culture results due to poor phlebotomy technique.
A. Improperly cleansed skin site
B. Improperly cleansed bottles
C. Neglecting to waste blood after drawing from a CVC (central venous catheter)
D. Failure to draw from multiple sites

A., B. and C. are all correct.

7.038 What is the purpose of the Allen test?
A. There is no such test
B. It evaluates the patient's platelet function
C. It evaluates the circulation in the radial artery
D. It evaluates the circulation in the ulnar artery

D. is the correct answer.

The Allen test is done prior to collection of blood from the radial artery for an arterial blood gas analysis. Oxygenated blood is supplied to the hand via the radial and ulnar arteries. The Allen test determines the ability of the ulnar artery to supply circulation to the hand. If the ulnar artery is not capable of supplying the area with blood, it is not advisable to puncture the radial artery. To perform the Allen test, both the radial and the ulnar arteries are compressed while the patient makes a fist. After the arm is dark red in color, the ulnar artery only is released. The hand should return to a pink color within 15 seconds. If it doesn't, this means that the ulnar artery is not capable of supplying blood to the hand and so the radial artery must not be punctured.

7.039 Which angle is the correct angle of the needle for an arterial draw?
A. 15°
B. 25°
C. 45°
D. 90°

C. is the correct answer.

7.040 When are arterial punctures used to collect blood?
A. When the patient doesn't have good veins
B. Some clinicians prefer to have their patients drawn by arterial puncture
C. At the patient's request
D. For arterial blood gases

D. is the correct answer.

7.041   Which of the following procedures should be followed when drawing arterial blood gases?
A. No tourniquet should be used
B. The patient should be fasting
C. The specimen must be transported at room temperature
D. All of the above

A. is the correct answer.

Additionally, the area should be cleansed with a povidone iodine type of cleanser.
No suction or back pressure on the syringe plunger is required since the syringe will self-fill due to high arterial blood pressure. Back pressure is to be avoided because it will alter the gas pressure of the sample. Vacutubes are to be avoided for the same reason.

7.042   Which of the following is important to remember to do after an arterial stick?
A. Greater pressure with a gauze pad should be applied to the puncture area than is necessary for venipuncture
B. The gauze pad should be applied with pressure for a maximum of 5 minutes
C. The gauze pad should be applied with pressure for at least 5–15 minutes
D. The arterial blood gas specimen should be transported on ice to the laboratory ASAP

A., C. and D. are all correct.

7.043   Which of the following are collected to monitor drug levels when the administration is continuous (IV drip, or to monitor patients whose basic medication levels have been established, but need to be periodically checked for correct dosage)?
A. Trough levels
B. Peak levels
C. Random levels
D. Daily levels

C. is the correct answer.

7.044   Which of the following will not affect how quickly a medication reaches its peak level in a patient?
A. The patient's metabolism
B. The type of medication
C. The mode of drug administration
D. The time of administration

D. is the correct answer.

7.045   If a test request that the personnel is unfamiliar with arrives in the laboratory, which of the following will provide all the information needed to correctly draw and run the test?
A. The Laboratory Procedure Manual
B. The MSDS sheets
C. OSHA's Bloodborne Pathogen Standard
D. The CDC

A. is the correct answer.

7.046   What protocols must a clinical laboratory follow in writing up their procedure manuals?
    A. The ASCP publishes a guideline that should be followed
    B. The Federal Register, which publishes rules and regulations governing clinical laboratories, requires that certain standards be met for setting procedure
    C. The clinical laboratory should obtain existing procedure manuals from other laboratories and follow their procedures
    D. All of the above

B. is the correct answer.

For details of the Federal Register that pertains to the rules and regulations governing the setting of procedure in clinical laboratories, see the Bibliography at the end of the Section.

7.047   Is it permissible to use a sample of blood that was originally collected for a CBC as a sample for a glycosylated hemoglobin (hemoglobin A_1C) test?
    A. Yes, since they both are collected in EDTA (lavender-topped) tubes
    B. No, since the glycosylated hemoglobin should have been refrigerated and the CBC probably wasn't refrigerated
    C. No, since the CBC was refrigerated and the glycosylated hemoglobin must not be refrigerated
    D. No, the two tests require entirely different anticoagulants

C. is the correct answer.

Both samples of blood should be collected in the lavender-topped, EDTA-preserved vacutube. However, CBCs are generally not put on ice or refrigerated immediately upon collection, and a glycosylated hemoglobin test should be collected this way. Therefore, a sample drawn originally for a CBC would not be suitable for glycosylated hemoglobin testing.

7.048   Is it permissible to use a sample of blood that was originally collected for a glycosylated hemoglobin (hemoglobin A_1C) test as a sample for a CBC?
    A. Yes, since they both are collected in EDTA (lavender-topped) tubes
    B. No, since the glycosylated hemoglobin should have been refrigerated, and the CBC probably wasn't refrigerated
    C. No, since the CBC was refrigerated and the glycosylated hemoglobin must not be refrigerated
    D. No, the two tests require entirely different anticoagulants

A. is the correct answer.

Refrigerated temperatures will not adversely affect the CBC, so it is permissible to use a sample originally intended for a glycosylated hemoglobin (hemoglobin A_1C) test for CBC analysis.

7.049   Can a sample of blood originally collected for a renin activity test be used for a glycosylated hemoglobin test?
    A. Yes, since both are collected in EDTA (lavender-topped) tubes
    B. No, since the blood for the renin activity test was not kept chilled, and the blood for a glycosylated hemoglobin test should have been chilled
    C. Yes, since both tests are collected in EDTA tubes and both are chilled
    D. No, since they require two entirely different anticoagulants

C. is the correct answer.

Blood collected for a renin activity test (helpful in diagnosing hypertension) should be drawn into a pre-chilled lavender-topped (EDTA-preserved) tube. The patient's blood is drawn into the pre-chilled tube and then immediately put back on ice. Because the blood is preserved with EDTA and chilled immediately, it is suitable for the glycosylated hemoglobin test.

7.050   Can a sample of blood originally collected for a renin activity test be used for a direct Coombs' test?
   A. Yes, since renin activities are collected in EDTA tubes, and direct Coombs' tests may be collected in this tube
   B. No, since the blood for the renin activity test is chilled, and the blood for a direct Coombs' test should not be chilled
   C. No, since the direct Coombs' test can only be done on serum, not plasma
   D. No, since they require two entirely different anticoagulants

A. is the correct answer.

The direct Coombs' test is a test performed in Immunohematology (Blood Bank) that tests for antibodies that are on the red blood cell, rather than in the serum or plasma. Usually, this can be done satisfactorily from serum obtained from a plain red-topped tube. Sometimes, however, a blood protein known as complement may interfere with the test. This happens when red blood cells become sensitized with complement and give a false-positive reaction to the Coombs' test. Complement can only do this in the presence of calcium so, in this case, blood must be used that lacks calcium. EDTA-preserved blood is used since the action of the EDTA preservative is to chelate calcium as a calcium–EDTA complex. In this case, the calcium ion is no longer available to activate complement. Chilling the EDTA-preserved specimen would not have a deleterious effect on the direct Coombs' test.

7.051   The PKU test is performed on:
   A. Newborns determined to be at risk
   B. All newborns
   C. Children before entering school
   D. People exhibiting symptoms

B. is the correct answer.

Phenylalanine is an amino acid that is normally metabolized to another amino acid called tyrosine. The enzyme phenylalaninehydroxylase facilitates this metabolic reaction. In phenylketonurics the action of the enzyme is blocked, with the result that phenylalanine is not converted to tyrosine. The result of this is a build-up of phenylalanine and its deaminated metabolites in the blood and spinal fluid. These products act as neurotoxins that can damage the nervous system, including the brain. Unless phenylketonurics follow a diet that is low in phenylalanine, mental retardation may result. For this reason, it is important to diagnose phenylketonurics very quickly after birth. When the child is 10 or 12 years old, the nervous system is generally well developed enough to withstand high levels of phenylalanine, and so a normal diet may be adopted.

7.052   The PKU test is performed:
    A. On serum collected in a plain red-topped tube
    B. On whole blood collected in a vacutube with a special anticoagulant
    C. On whole blood collected in drops on a special blotting paper
    D. On sweat collected with a special apparatus that induces sweating

C. is the correct answer.

To collect blood for the PKU test, five drops of blood are collected from a neonate onto a special blotting paper for PKU testing that is sent to a reference laboratory for testing. The blotting paper contains five printed circles which should each receive a drop of blood from the infant. The blood will be tested for the presence of tyrosine, which indicates normal metabolism of phenylalanine. The drops of blood must be fairly precise in their size. They must be neither so large that they extend beyond the perimeters of the circles on the blotting paper, nor must they be so small that they fail to fill the area circumscribed by the circles. As with any skin puncture, the first drop of blood should be wiped away with a sterile gauze pad, before subsequent drops are collected for analysis.

7.053   What is the purpose of the sweat chloride test?
    A. To test for phenylketonuria
    B. To test for porphyrins
    C. To screen for cystic fibrosis
    D. To screen for muscular dystrophy

C. is the correct answer.

The sweat chloride test is performed to screen for cystic fibrosis (CF).
CF is a disorder of the exocrine glands that produce mucus, sweat and saliva. There is an increase in the amount of mucus in the lungs, making it difficult for people with cystic fibrosis to breathe. People with CF produce chloride in their perspiration that is 2–5 times the normal production, and it is this high chloride that is measured and used to screen for cystic fibrosis.

7.054   How is the sweat chloride test performed?
    A. It is performed on blood collected without anticoagulants
    B. It is performed on blood collected with a special anticoagulant
    C. It is performed on sweat collected with an apparatus designed to produce sweat
    D. It is performed on sputum obtained from a productive cough

C. is the correct answer.

To perform the sweat chloride test, the patient must be induced to produce sweat. The sweat is collected onto pre-weighed gauze pads and then analyzed for chloride content. To induce the patient to sweat, an alkaloid called pilocarpine hydrochloric acid is applied to a gauze pad and placed on the patient's skin. A low electrical current is then applied which draws the pilocarpine into the skin by iontophoresis. The pilocarpine induces the sweat glands to secrete profusely.

7.055   When collecting blood for the cold agglutinin test:
  A. The blood should be collected in a pre-chilled plain red-topped tube
  B. The blood should be collected in a plain red-topped tube and then should be put on ice
  C. The blood must not be allowed to clot; collect in a tube with EDTA anticoagulant
  D. The blood must be allowed to clot at body temperature

D. is the correct answer.

Ideally, blood collected for the cold agglutinin test should be allowed to clot at body temperature, which is 37 ℃. To collect a specimen properly, a red-stoppered tube should be placed in a 37 ℃ incubator 30 minutes before the collection is to be done. A portable incubator should then be employed to transport the pre-warmed tube to the patient. After the specimen has been drawn, the tube should be returned to the portable incubator, and sent to the laboratory. In the lab, the blood should be centrifuged in a 37 ℃ warm room or else in a heated, jacketed centrifuge.

7.056   Which of the following tests determines platelet function?
  A. Ivy bleeding time test
  B. Prothrombin test
  C. Fibrinogen test
  D. Partial thromboplastin test

A. is the correct answer.

The bleeding time test establishes how long it takes a patient to stop bleeding on his/her own after a standardized incision has been made. The bleeding time test is a useful tool for testing platelet plug formation in the capillaries. Platelets are the first blood component to come to the site of vessel damage. They begin to clump together to form the platelet plug, which is the first step in forming a blood clot. Platelets with normal activity have this ability to clump together into the platelet plug. Bleeding times assess platelet numbers and function. Abnormally low numbers of plts will cause a bleeding time to be prolonged because there simply aren't enough platelets to form the plug. Also, platelets possessing abnormal activity will not be able to form a plug properly, and may exhibit bleeding problems.

7.057   When a bleeding time test is performed, where is the best location to make the standardized incision?
  A. At the end of the 3rd or 4th digit, on the side
  B. Lateral to imaginary lines drawn from the center of the heel to the great toe and from the heel to the 5th toe
  C. On the earlobe
  D. Over the lateral volar surface of the forearm, approximately 5 cm below the antecubital crease

D. is the correct answer.

The procedure is best performed over the lateral volar surface of the forearm, approximately 5 cm below the antecubital crease. Avoid surface veins, scars, bruises and edematous areas in order to obtain accurate results.

7.058   Which of the following blades is used to make the standardized incision of the bleeding time test?
   A. A surgical scalpel
   B. A Surgicutt device
   C. An Autolet device
   D. A pediatric lancet

B. is the correct answer.

The Surgicutt instrument will come with a safety clip which should be removed. Hold the device securely between the thumb and middle finger. Gently rest it on the patient's forearm and apply minimal pressure so that both ends of the Surgicutt are lightly touching the patient's skin. Do not press down so hard that a very deep incision is created. Conversely, do not allow the Surgicutt to barely touch the skin resulting in an incision that is too shallow. By holding the Surgicutt evenly, it is ensured that neither end of the incision is deeper than the other. A horizontal incision parallel to the antecubital crease is then made by pressing the trigger of the Surgicutt to spring the blade.

7.059   What is the pressure that the blood pressure cuff (sphygmomanometer) should be inflated to for a bleeding time test?
   A. Equal to the patient's systolic blood pressure reading
   B. Equal to the patient's diastolic blood pressure reading
   C. 40 pounds of pressure
   D. A sphygmomanometer is not used for a bleeding time test

C. is the correct answer.

Prior to making the incision for the bleeding time test, place the blood pressure cuff on the upper arm. Inflate the cuff to 40 mmHg. Hold at this pressure for the duration of the test.

7.060   What is the purpose of the filter paper that is used during a bleeding time test?
   A. It is used to collect drops of blood that will be analyzed in the laboratory
   B. It is used to wick away blood that appears at the incision site
   C. It is used to filter the reagents that are used in the test
   D. Filter paper is not used during a bleeding time test

B. is the correct answer.

The Surgicutt should be gently depressed, and simultaneously a stopwatch should be started. The blade will make an incision 5 mm long by 1 mm deep. After 30 seconds, wick the flow of blood with filter paper. Bring the filter paper close to the incision, but do not touch the paper directly onto the incision, so as not to disturb the formation of a platelet plug. Wick the blood away every 30 seconds thereafter until blood no longer stains the paper. Stop the timer, which will now reflect the bleeding time. The normal range (NR) will vary somewhat with the brand of Surgicutt device used, but your institution will have its own protocol and NR established. Typically, the NR is between 2 and 8 minutes.

7.061   A patient scheduled for a bleeding time test should refrain from which of the following for 7–10 days prior to the test?
   A. Food
   B. Alcohol
   C. Caffeine
   D. Aspirin

B. and D. are the correct answers.

Since aspirin interferes with the platelet's ability to function normally, the patient should refrain from the use of aspirin or aspirin-containing products for 7–10 days prior to the test. There are some other substances, most notably alcohol, that can cause a prolonged BT.

7.062　The condition in which all the cellular elements of the blood are increased is known as:
A. Leukemia
B. Leukopenia
C. Thrombocytopenia
D. Polycythemia

D. is the correct answer.

7.063　A therapeutic phlebotomy is:
A. The removal of a large quantity (usually about 1000 ml) of the patient's blood
B. Used to treat polycythemia
C. Used to goad the bone marrow into producing more blood cells
D. Any phlebotomy procedure is a therapeutic phlebotomy procedure

A. and B. are the correct answers.

All the cellular elements of the blood of patients with polycythemia are increased. If not monitored, these patients are at increased risk of stroke and heart attack. These patients come to the health-care institution responsible for their care on a regular basis to have some of their blood removed by means of a therapeutic phlebotomy.
Special therapeutic phlebotomy bottles are utilized. These are very much like giant evacuated tubes. They contain an anticoagulant and hold about 1000 ml of blood. There is a needle assembly with long tubing that is also connected to a rubber stopper in the bottle. The patient is drawn lying down since such a large amount of blood is being removed.

Bibliography

Federal Register. published Friday, February 28, 1992;57(No. 40):7164

American Association of Blood Banks Technical Manual. Philadelphia, Toronto: J.B. Lippincott Company, 1981

NCCLS Specimen Collection. *Procedures for the Collection of Diagnostic Blood Specimens by Venipuncture*. NCCLS Document H3-A3, Vol. 11, No. 10, July 1991

NCCLS Specimen Collection. *Percutaneous Collection of Arterial Blood for Laboratory Analysis*. NCCLS Document H11-A, Vol. 5, No. 3, April 1985

NCCLS Specimen Collection. *Collection and Transportation of Single Collection Urine Specimens*. NCCLS Document GP8-P, Vol. 5, No. 7, May 1985

NCCLS Specimen Collection. *Collection and Preservation of Timed Urine Specimens*. NCCLS Document GP13-P, Vol. 7, No. 8, September 1987

One touch II, blood glucose monitoring system. *Manual and Inservice Guide for Hospitals and Clinics*. Milpitas, CA: Lifescan, a Johnson & Johnson Co., March 1991

BBL Vacutainer Brand. *Culture Bottles For Blood Cultures*. Revised edn. Package Insert 88-1185-2. Cockeysville, MD: Becton Dickinson Microbiology Systems, October 1993

ALBA's Medical Technology. Board Examination Review. 9th edn. Anaheim, CA: A Berkeley Scientific Publication, 1951

Bailey and Scott's Diagnostic Microbiology. St. Louis, Toronto, London: The C.V. Mosby Company, 1982

Garza D, Becan-McBride K. *Phlebotomy Handbook*. 3rd edn. Norwalk, CT: Appleton and Lange, 1993

SECTION 8:   QUALITY CONTROL

Objectives

- To be able to describe the method used to assure accuracy in drawing blood
- To be able to describe methods of QA in equipment and supplies

Key facts

A.   Quality assurance in blood collection
    1.   Appropriate patient preparation
        a.   Fasting, if appropriate
        b.   Accurate ID
        c.   Timed specimens drawn at correct time
        d.   Appropriate specimen container used (with appropriate anticoagulant)
        e.   Appropriate transport and storage
        f.   Specimen not hemolyzed, drawn short or in any other way unsatisfactory
        g.   Documentation log kept for:
            1.   Unsuccessful venipunctures
            2.   Patient refusal
            3.   Patient unavailability
            4.   + and – blood culture log kept for purposes of tracking contamination

B.   Quality assurance in equipment maintenance and supplies
    1.   Expiration dates checked
    2.   Tubes from each lot number checked for:
        a.   Vacuum draw
        b.   Anticoagulant viability
        c.   Sterility
        d.   Integrity during centrifugation
    3.   Equipment maintenance
        a.   Daily controls
        b.   Monthly calibration
        c.   Centrifuge speed checks
        d.   Daily temperatures recorded; thermometers calibrated quarterly

C.   Quality assurance in transport
    1.   Integrity of sample maintained
        a.   Federal regulations regarding shipping biohazardous material

D.   Quality control management
    1.   TQM
    2.   CQI

Questions and Answers

8.001 Which of the following concepts are concerned with continually striving to increase customer satisfaction?
A. TQM
B. CQI
C. TDM
D. QC

A. and B. are the correct answers.

TQM is an acronym for total quality management and CQI is an acronym for continuous quality improvement. Basically these two concepts are identical, the goal of both is to strive continually in order to increase customer satisfaction.

8.002 Which of the following are not among the steps involved in improving the quality of a service?
A. Identify problems
B. Propose solutions
C. Experiment
D. Implement changes

C. is the correct answer.

The basic steps that are involved in improving the quality of a service are as follows:
a. Outline the process;
b. Collect data;
c. Identify problems;
d. Propose solutions;
e. Implement changes.

8.003 Which of the following organizations provides accreditation to clinical laboratories that have appropriate quality control procedures in place? These clinical laboratories must implement these procedures in a manner acceptable to standards.
A. CAP
B. OSHA
C. JCAHO
D. ASCP

A. is the correct answer.

CAP stands for the College of American Pathologists. The CAP provides accreditation to clinical laboratories that have appropriate quality control procedures in place and that implement these procedures in a manner acceptable to CAP standards.

8.004 Which of the following organizations issues policies concerned with employee safety?
A. CAP
B. OSHA
C. JCAHO
D. ASCP

B. is the correct answer.

OSHA stands for Occupational Safety and Health Administration. This organization issues policies concerned with employee safety.

8.005 Which of the following organizations is concerned with improving the quality of care provided by organized health-care facilities?
A. CAP
B. OSHA
C. JCAHO
D. ASCP

C. is the correct answer.

JCAHO is the acronym for the Joint Commission on the Accreditation of Healthcare Organizations. JCAHO was established in 1951. It is a private, non-profit-making organization concerned with improving the quality of care provided by organized health-care facilities. JCAHO offers accreditation to health-care organizations in the United States that are able to meet its standards for quality care.

8.006   Which of the following is a professional organization that provides certification to laboratory professionals?
   A. CAP
   B. OSHA
   C. JCAHO
   D. ASCP

D. is the correct answer.

ASCP stands for the American Society of Clinical Pathologists. It is one of the professional organizations that provides certification to qualified clinical laboratory professionals such as medical technologists, medical laboratory technicians, histotechnologists, cytotechnologists and phlebotomists.

8.007   TQM and CQI programs stress the need for constant education and training. What level of employees are believed to benefit most from continuing education?
   A. Laboratory support personnel such as phlebotomists and laboratory assistants
   B. Laboratory staff who perform the bench work, such as medical technologists and medical laboratory technicians
   C. Department supervisors
   D. Every employee of the health-care facility from top management down

D. is the correct answer.

8.008   TQM and CQI programs are:
   A. Universal for all businesses
   B. Applicable for all businesses with modifications for each business
   C. Designed specifically for businesses involved in health care
   D. None of the above

B. is the correct answer.

8.009   What are some quality assurance issues concerning sample collection?
   A. The patient should be prepared properly for the test; this means that the patient should be fasting if necessary and medications withheld if necessary
   B. The patient should be identified accurately prior to the sample collection
   C. The appropriate blood collection tubes (anticoagulant, non-anticoagulant) should be used for blood collection
   D. All of the above

D. is the correct answer.

Additionally, the sample should be collected at the appropriate time and the sample should be acceptable for testing, (quantity sufficient, not hemolyzed, etc.).

8.010   What kind of quality assurance issues are there involving transport and storage of samples?
   A. The conditions of transport must be appropriate for that sample
   B. The sample must be transported to the testing laboratory in a timely manner
   C. Once the samples have arrived at the laboratory, they must be stored appropriately
   D. All of the above

D. is the correct answer.

Appropriate conditions of transport may include protection from light, chilled temperatures, room temperatures or incubation at body temperature when appropriate.
Timelines of transport can be monitored by writing the time drawn on the tube, and then logging the time received in the laboratory.
Upon arrival at the laboratory, if the samples are not to undergo testing immediately, they must be stored under their optimal conditions of preservation.

8.011   What does stock rotation involve?
   A. Laboratory supplies should be organized so that only one lot number is used at a time
   B. Laboratory supplies should be intermingled, to avoid using only one lot number
   C. Laboratory supplies should be arranged so that those with expiration dates that will outdate first are taken off the shelf first
   D. Laboratory supplies should be stored in the order in which they arrive in the laboratory

C. is the correct answer.

The expiration dates must be checked on new shipments, and shelves stocked so that tubes that outdate first are taken off the shelf first. When restocking their own trays, collectors should check the expiration dates on the tubes they are using for restocking, to be sure that they are not outdated.

8.012   Which of the following tests should be performed on a newly arrived supply of vacutubes?
   A. Several tubes from each new shipment should be tested for vacuum draw
   B. Anticoagulant ability should be tested
   C. Sterility
   D. Integrity during centrifugation

A., B., C. and D. are all correct.

Several tubes from each new shipment should be tested for vacuum draw. This can be done by using a needle, needle holder and a beaker of water. The needle and needle holder are assembled as usual. The uncapped needle is submerged in a beaker of water, and several tubes from the lot are pushed onto the needle assembly. If the vacuum draw is appropriate, the tube will fill with water.
The ability of the anticoagulant to prevent clot formation should also be tested on each new lot shipment. Blood is drawn into a tube and inverted, and then the blood is strained through gauze to check for clots.
Tubes should be sterile, and can be tested by the Microbiology department.
Integrity during centrifugation can be tested also. During this check, a vacutainer serum-separator tube filled with a blood sample is utilized. A good centrifugation spindown will be observed when the serum separator migrates to the level between the cellular and serum components of the blood sample.

8.013   One of the job responsibilities of the phlebotomist at a certain hospital is to record daily the temperatures of the laboratory's several refrigerators, incubators, heat blocks and room temperatures. How can the hospital be assured that the recorded temperatures are really the true temperatures?
   A. By using only NBS (National Bureau of Standards) certified thermometers
   B. By calibrating the thermometers used against an NBS (National Bureau of Standards) certified thermometer on a quarterly basis
   C. By using at least two thermometers for each check
   D. None of the above

B. is the correct answer.

8.014   When performing a quality control check on a sphygmomanometer (used in the laboratory for BT testing), the sphygmomanometer gauge is checked for accuracy against a 'calibrating gauge'. How closely should the two gauges read?
A. There should not be a difference of more than 2 mmHg
B. There should not be a difference of more than 5 mmHg
C. There should not be a difference of more than 10 mmHg
D. Any difference at all is unacceptable

B. is the correct answer.

8.015   What centrifugal or *g* force is generally necessary for good separation of the cellular components from the serum or plasma?
A. 500 for 10 minutes
B. 3500 for 10 minutes
C. 1000 for 10 minutes
D. 10 000 for 10 minutes

C. is the correct answer.

8.016   In order to check a centrifuge for accurate speed, a tachometer is used to determine the centrifuge's ______________. This information is used to calculate the *g* force.
A. Speed
B. Revolutions per minute (RPMs)
C. Centrifugal force
D. Decibels

B. is the correct answer.

The speed of the centrifuges used in the laboratory should be checked monthly. A tachometer is used to evaluate the RPMs (revolutions per minute). The centrifugal force or the *g* value is then calculated. A *g* force of 1000 for 10 minutes is usually sufficient for good separation of cells from serum or plasma. (Follow manufacturer's directives on this.)

8.017   Which of the following reagents mimic patient samples, except that because they are manufactured, the concentration of their analytes is known?
A. Controls
B. Calibrators
C. Diluents
D. Specimens

A. is the correct answer.

The instrumentation used in a laboratory must be subjected to regular quality control checks. One way in which the integrity of the instruments is checked is with the use of manufactured control serum containing a known amount of analyte(s). Controls are run under exactly the same testing conditions as the patient samples. The manufacturer establishes what the concentration of a particular analyte in the control is, and then establishes a range of acceptability, (normally 2 standard deviations above and below the mean concentration of the analyte). The instrument must be able to achieve results that are within this range of acceptability in order to meet quality assurance requirements.

8.018   Which of the following quality control reagents set the baseline readings of the laboratory testing instruments?
A. Controls
B. Calibrators
C. Diluents
D. Specimens

B. is the correct answer.

Like controls, calibrators contain known amounts of analytes, but in this case they are used to set the instrument's internal parameters against which all subsequent samples (including controls) will be measured. For example, a glucose calibrator may contain 100 g of glucose/dl. The calibrator is introduced to the instrument and the instrument is told that this sample contains 100 g of glucose/dl. All subsequent samples introduced to the instrument are compared to the calibrator which contained 100 g of glucose/dl, and comparisons are made. Based on these comparisons, the instrument determines the concentration of glucose in all subsequent samples introduced to it.

8.019   What is 'standard deviation'?
A. The amount of deviation from a true result that is allowable
B. A statistical expression for reporting the amount of variance in measurements
C. Precision
D. Accuracy

B. is the correct answer.

When several readings concerning the concentration of a substance are obtained, there is going to be a small amount of variance between the results. Standard deviation is a statistical expression for reporting the amount of variance. If there was no variance in the measurements, the standard deviation would be zero. Standard deviation is used to set up limits of acceptable variance in the results obtained when determining the concentration of an analyte in a substance.

8.020   Which of the following tests should be performed prior to an arterial puncture?
A. A CBC
B. Electrolytes
C. A BT (bleeding time) test
D. The Allen test

D. is the correct answer.

Collateral circulation is the circulation provided to an area by alternative blood vessels, other than the one to be used for obtaining a blood sample. When utilizing the radial artery for an arterial puncture, the collector should first determine that the ulnar artery will provide the hand with sufficient circulation. The Allen test is performed to ensure that the ulnar artery is capable of doing this, and, in this manner, is a quality assurance check for arterial blood gas puncture.

Bibliography

TQM, Reengineering, and the Edge of Chaos. Quality Progress. February 1996

Clinical Laboratory Science. The Journal of the American Society for Medical Technologists. Mar/Apr 1993. Vol. 6, No. 6. McEnerney K. Quality teams: the foundation of quality improvement. *Clin Lab Sci* 1993; 6

URL: http//www.nnlm.nlm.nih.gov/nnlm/jcaho.html

Neter J, Wasserman W, Whitmore G. *Applied Statistics*. 3rd edn. Newton, MA: Allyn and Bacon, 1988

NCCLS Specimen Collection. *Percutaneous Collection of Arterial Blood for Laboratory Analysis*. NCCLS Document H11-A, Vol. 5, No. 3, April 1985

SECTION 9:   INTERPERSONAL SKILLS

Objectives

- To be able to prepare a patient for laboratory testing
- To be familiar with the major points of the Patients' Bill of Rights
- To be able to identify important communication skills
- To be aware of barriers to good communication

Key facts

A.   Patients' Bill of Rights

B.   Communication
   1.   Verbal
   2.   Non-verbal
   3.   Listening skills

C.   Other interpersonal skills
   1.   Appearance
   2.   Ethics
   3.   Responsibilities

Questions and Answers

9.001   A patient's confidentiality is guaranteed to them by which of the following?
   A. JCAHO's 10-Step Process of the Monitoring and Evaluation Process
   B. AHA's Patients' Bill of Rights
   C. Continuous Quality Improvement
   D. CLIA '88

B. is the correct answer.

Most health-care facilities have incorporated a Patients' Bill of Rights into their health-care policy. Usually these Patients' Bill of Rights are based on the American Hospital Association's Patients' Bill of Rights that were approved in 1973. The purpose of a Patients' Bill of Rights is to enable the patients to at least be cognizant of, and perhaps be participatory contributors to, their own health care.

9.002   The breach of patient confidentiality by a health-care employee can result in:
   A. A verbal warning by the employer
   B. A written warning by the employer
   C. Instant dismissal from the job
   D. No formal punitive action, but health-care personnel should refrain from this

C. is the correct answer.

One of the most important parts of any Patients' Bill of Rights policy is the guarantee of patient confidentiality. Employees who are actively involved in the care of a patient may discuss the pertinent facts of the patient's health history in carrying out their health-care duties, but great discretion must be practiced to prevent inappropriate people from participating in the exchange of information.

9.003   How should a collector respond when a patient asks for the results of previously drawn tests?
   A. The collector should refer the question to the clinician in charge of the patient's care
   B. The collector should use discretion, if the results are not alarming it is permissible to convey them to the patient.
   C. The collector should ignore the patient
   D. The collector should rebuke the patient for asking an inappropriate question

A. is the correct answer.

A proviso of almost any Patients' Bill of Rights stipulates that physicians and perhaps some other authorized personnel should be the only people who may give patients the results of their health-care procedures and explain the meaning of the test results. For unauthorized personnel to do this may be cause for dismissal. The phlebotomist should explain this briefly to the patient who is requesting the information.

9.004   How should a phlebotomist respond when a patient refuses to allow his/her blood to be drawn?
   A. The phlebotomist should explain that the patient must allow the testing, that the patient signed away the right to refuse treatment upon admission
   B. The phlebotomist could acknowledge the patient's right to refuse treatment but point out that the clinician ordered the tests for a reason
   C. The phlebotomist should not waste time arguing with the patient, make a note of the refusal and allow the clinician to deal with it
   D. The phlebotomist should get some help if necessary, and draw the blood anyway

B. is the correct answer.

The right to refuse treatment is guaranteed to patients under the Patients' Bill of Rights. The phlebotomist can acknowledge that the patient has the right to refuse treatment, but should try not to accept the patient's decision too eagerly. Pointing out that the patient's physician has ordered these tests for a reason, to help diagnose the patient's problem and to help the physician plan treatment may convince the patient to allow the testing.

9.005   Which of the following rights is guaranteed in most
Patients' Bill of Rights?
A. The right to know the identification of all
personnel involved in the patient's care
B. The right to know if the health-care facility's staff
includes students
C. Neither of the above is a guaranteed patient right
D. Both A. and B. are rights guaranteed to patients

D. is the correct answer.

9.006   Which of the following is generally not a right
guaranteed to patients by the Patients' Bill of
Rights?
A. The patient has the right to be treated
courteously during his care
B. The patient has the right to receive all
information about his health status necessary to
make informed decisions
C. The patient has the right to be informed of the
availability of generic drugs that may be used in
his treatment
D. The patient has the right to information about all
procedures done on his behalf. If the patient
requests information about alternative
procedures, this must also be provided

C. is the correct answer.

Although patients should be informed as to the
availability of generic drugs, it is not a guaranteed
right under most Patients' Bill of Rights.

9.007   Which of the following rights is guaranteed to
patients by the Patients' Bill of Rights?
A. When a patient's clinician requests a consultation
with another clinician, the patient has a right to
know
B. The health-care facility where the patient has
sought care will provide that care to the best of
its ability, and will inform the patient if his
situation can be better met at an alternative
health-care facility, provided the alternative site
has accepted the patient
C. The patient has a right to be informed if his/her
care will involve scientific experimentation; the
patient has the right to refuse to allow any
physical substances obtained in his/her care to be
released for scientific experimentation
D. All of the above

D. is the correct answer.

9.008   Which of the following rights are guaranteed to
patients by the Patients' Bill of Rights?
A. The patient has the right to see all bills in
connection with treatment, and to have them
explained
B. The patient has a right to know what rules apply
to the patient, such as not eating when the test
requires a fasting specimen
C. The patient's demographic data should be
treated in a confidential manner
D. All of the above

D. is the correct answer.

9.009   While preparing to draw a patient's blood for testing, the collector is questioned by the patient as to what tests are being done, and why each test is being done. How should the collector respond to these queries?
  A. The collector should refer the questions to the clinician in charge of the patient's care
  B. The collector may briefly describe the reasons for the tests ordered
  C. The collector should reply that s/he doesn't know, s/he only collects the blood
  D. The collector should ignore such questions

B. is the correct answer.

Although only physicians and authorized personnel may give a patient test results, and explain the meaning of the results, it is permissible for ancillary health-care providers to briefly describe to a patient what procedures are being performed. Without providing information that may be alarming to the patient, brief explanations as to why procedures are being done may be given also.

9.010   A phlebotomist is asked by a patient for some assistance in changing position in bed, since the patient is feeling uncomfortable and cramped. How should the phlebotomist handle this request?
  A. The phlebotomist should refuse since this is a nursing responsibility
  B. The phlebotomist should comply since the patient is the customer
  C. The phlebotomist should inform the patient that s/he must change positions by her/himself
  D. The phlebotomist should offer to obtain nursing help for the patient

A. and D. are the correct answers.

Some requests by patients are better carried out by nursing personnel, and should not be handled by ancillary staff. Nursing personnel are more informed about a patient's specific needs and restrictions, and are better able to make informed decisions. For example, certain movements and positions may be contraindicated, depending on the patient's condition. When these requests are made, it is better to offer to bring the request to the attention of nursing personnel, than to comply with the request itself.

9.011   Why is it inappropriate for ancillary staff to comply with a patient's request for food and/or drink?
  A. The food and/or drink may be contraindicated
  B. Ancillary personnel don't know where such items are kept
  C. All hospital employees are very busy, and should only perform their specific duties
  D. All of the above

A. is the correct answer.

Nursing personnel are more informed about a patient's specific needs and restrictions, and are better able to make informed decisions.

9.012   Why is it inappropriate for phlebotomists to comply with a patient's request for the phlebotomist to empty the patient's bedpan?
  A. The phlebotomist is not properly trained to perform this function
  B. The contents may be needed for analysis, and the phlebotomist may not be aware of this
  C. It probably is all right for the phlebotomist to perform this task for the patient
  D. None of the above

B. is the correct answer.

Nursing personnel are more informed about a patient's specific needs and restrictions, and are better able to make informed decisions.

9.013   Which of the following is probably the best technique to help ensure good communication?
  A. Consciously listen intently
  B. The listener should repeat what the speaker says so that both parties are reassured of good communication
  C. Stop all other activities when being spoken to
  D. Stand up when being spoken to

B. is the correct answer.

Although all of the suggestions are good ones, the single best method that reassures both parties that good communication is taking place is for the participants of a conversation to repeat what the other says. Miscommunications are instantly known to the communicators in this way.

9.014   Which of the following is the appropriate way to communicate with the public in a health-care setting?
   A.   Use specific medical and scientific terminology so that the patient will be reassured that you are professional and knowledgeable
   B.   Avoid using specific medical and scientific terminology that the patient won't understand
   C.   Be as non-committal as possible; it is the function of the clinician to communicate with the patient
   D.   None of the above

B. is the correct answer.

Collectors dealing with the public should try to avoid using medical and scientific terminology that lay people are not familiar with. Patients are often nervous and uncertain about procedures being done to them, and incomprehensible language by the health-care providers will exacerbate these feelings.
Often, patients for medical procedures are elderly. They may be confused and/or hard of hearing. Collectors should take the extra time and effort necessary to communicate clearly with these patients.
Collectors should always strive to be professional and courteous, both to the patients and to colleagues.

9.015   Which of the following will probably not enhance your listening skills?
   A.   If someone begins to speak to you while you are in the middle of a task, you should turn to them as soon as possible and tell them that you weren't able to concentrate on what they were saying, and ask them to begin again
   B.   To ensure that you are concentrating on what a person is saying, and also to be sure that the person you are speaking to is concentrating on you, establish eye contact
   C.   When someone is speaking to you, provide them with verbal feedback so that they can sense whether or not their message was interpreted properly; this also provides you with assurance that you heard the message correctly
   D.   Attempt to do several things at once to train yourself in the co-ordination of tasks

D. is the correct answer.

9.016   What is non-verbal communication?
   A.   The use of facial expression, posture, gestures and appearance to convey ideas
   B.   To be non-communicative
   C.   The projection of ideas, thoughts or feelings without spoken words
   D.   The projection of ideas, thoughts or feelings with spoken words

A. and C. are the correct answers.

9.017   According to some experts, how large a part of our communication is due to our 'body language'?
A. 10%
B. 20%
C. 50%
D. 90%

C. is the correct answer.

It is important to project a positive image through body language when dealing with the public. Health-care providers may find themselves in situations that they feel apprehensive about. A little hesitancy is natural, but health-care providers should try not to alarm the patient with their own apprehension. If the situation seems overwhelming, the health-care provider should obtain some assistance. Health-care providers may also find themselves in situations that try their patience. Again, they should avoid body language that projects their sense of exasperation, and try to deal calmly and courteously with the patient.

9.018   Which of the following contribute to projecting an image of intelligence and competence?
A. Erect posture
B. Clean hands and fingernails
C. Clean and neat clothing
D. A courteous manner

A., B., C. and D. are all correct answers.

Most clinical centers will have a dress code for employees. In general, employees in health-care situations should attempt to be well groomed and clean. By its nature, health-care work entails fairly intimate contact with strangers; for reasons of sanitation and because of the confidence it inspires, health-care workers should employ high standards of cleanliness. Health-care employees should remember that not only they, but also the institutions that they represent, are being judged by the patients.

9.019   Which members of the health-care team take the Hippocratic Oath?
A. Physicians
B. Clinicians (physicians, physician assistants, nurse practitioners)
C. Clinicians and all ancillary staff
D. None of the above

A. is the correct answer.

Only physicians take the Hippocratic Oath, but remember that originally physicians performed all the tasks that are now dispersed among ancillary staff. Therefore, the standards of behavior of the Hippocratic Oath are meant to apply to every member of the health-care team.

9.020   Which of the following is a tenant of the Hippocratic Oath?
A. To do no harm to anyone intentionally
B. To perform according to your best judgment
C. Not to attempt to do something beyond your training and knowledge
D. All of the above

D. is the correct answer.

Two additional tenants of the Hippocratic Oath are, first, to restrict your activities to those patients who have been assigned to you, in order to avoid getting involved with patients out of curiosity, and, second, to adhere strictly to patient confidentiality.

9.021   Which of the following is not a responsibility of the phlebotomist?
   A. Practicing courtesy to patients and to colleagues
   B. Taking care to obtain appropriate samples from correct patients in a timely manner
   C. Transporting specimens appropriately
   D. Giving patients sovereign remedies for their ailments

D. is the correct answer.

It's actually illegal to practice medicine without a license.

9.022   A phlebotomist who has completed an approved phlebotomy course at a local community college and passed the national certification exam is trained to do a procedure differently on his first job than he learned in the course. The phlebotomist should:
   A. Observe the collection procedures of the institution that employs him/her even if they are contradictory to procedures learned elsewhere
   B. Refuse to do the procedure differently than it was presented in the approved course
   C. Report the community college to the certifying agency
   D. Report the place of employment to the certifying agency

A. is the correct answer.

There may be more than one correct way of doing a procedure. All clinical health facilities should have procedure manuals outlining every procedure done at that facility. These procedure manuals are reviewed by one or several agencies on a regular basis.

9.023   From which of the following should the phlebotomist refrain?
   A. Discussions concerning a patient's ailments with the patient
   B. Evaluating the therapies assigned to the patient
   C. Discussion and evaluation of physicians and other colleagues with the patient
   D. All of the above

D. is the correct answer.

9.024   JCAHO has a 10-Step Process that emphasizes continuous improvement of health care provided to the public. What is the 1st step in this 10-step process concerned with?
   A. Delineation of the scope of care and service to the patient
   B. Assigning of responsibility among health-care professionals
   C. Identification of the important aspects of care and service
   D. Identification of indicators for the important aspects of care and service

B. is the correct answer.

JCAHO's 10-Step Process:
Step 1. Assign responsibility:
   a. Involve organization leaders;
   b. Design and foster approach to continuous improvement of quality;
   c. Set priorities for assessment and improvement.

9.025   JCAHO has a 10-Step Process that emphasizes continuous improvement of health care provided to the public. What is the 2nd step in this 10-step process concerned with?
- A. Delineation of the scope of care and service to the patient
- B. Assigning of responsibility among health-care professionals
- C. Identification of the important aspects of care and service
- D. Identification of indicators for the important aspects of care and service

A. is the correct answer.

JCAHO's 10-Step Process:
Step 2. Delineate the scope of care and service:
- a. Identify the functions and/or identify the procedures, treatments and other activities performed in the organization.

9.026   JCAHO has a 10-Step Process that emphasizes continuous improvement of health care provided to the public. What is the 3rd step in this 10-step process concerned with?
- A. Delineation of the scope of care and service to the patient
- B. Assigning of responsibility among health-care professionals
- C. Identification of the important aspects of care and service
- D. Identification of indicators for the important aspects of care and service

C. is the correct answer.

JCAHO's 10-Step Process:
Step 3. Identify important aspects of care and service:
- a. Determine the key functions, treatments, processes, and other aspects of care and service that warrant ongoing monitoring;
- b. Establish priorities among the important aspects of care and service chosen.

9.027   JCAHO has a 10-Step Process that emphasizes continuous improvement of health care provided to the public. What is the 4th step in this 10-step process concerned with?
- A. Delineation of the scope of care and service to the patient
- B. Assigning of responsibility among health-care professionals
- C. Identification of the important aspects of care and service
- D. Identification of indicators for the important aspects of care and service

D. is the correct answer.

JCAHO's 10-Step Process:
Step 4. Identify indicators:
- a. Identify teams to develop indicators for the important aspects of care and service;
- b. Select indicators.

9.028   JCAHO has a 10-Step Process that emphasizes continuous improvement of health care provided to the public. What is the 5th step in this 10-step process concerned with?
- A. Establishing thresholds for evaluation
- B. Collecting and organizing data
- C. Initiating evaluation
- D. Taking actions to improve care and service

A. is the correct answer.

JCAHO's 10-Step Process:
Step 5. Establish thresholds for evaluation:
- a. Each team identifies thresholds for each indicator;
- b. Select thresholds.

9.029   JCAHO has a 10-Step Process that emphasizes continuous improvement of health care provided to the public. What is the 6th step in this 10-step process concerned with?
A. Establishing thresholds for evaluation
B. Collecting and organizing data
C. Initiating evaluation
D. Taking actions to improve care and service

B. is the correct answer.

JCAHO's 10-Step Process:
Step 6. Collect and organize data:
a. Each team identifies data sources and data-collection methods for the recommended indicators;
b. The data-collection methodology is designed, and those responsible for collection, organization and applying thresholds are identified;
c. Collect data;
d. Organize data so thresholds for evaluation can be applied;
e. Collect data so thresholds for evaluation can be applied;
f. Collect data from other sources, including patient and staff surveys, comments, suggestions and complaints.

9.030   JCAHO has a 10-Step Process that emphasizes continuous improvement of health care provided to the public. What is the 7th step in this 10-step process concerned with?
A. Establishing thresholds for evaluation
B. Collecting and organizing data
C. Initiating evaluation
D. Taking actions to improve care and service

C. is the correct answer.

JCAHO's 10-Step Process:
Step 7. Initiate evaluation:
a. Apply thresholds of evaluation to indicator data;
b. Initiate evaluation of aspect of care or service if threshold is reached;
c. Assess other feedback (for example, staff suggestions, patient satisfaction survey results) that may contribute to priority setting for evaluation;
d. Set priorities for evaluation;
e. Teams undertake intensive evaluation.

9.031   JCAHO has a 10-Step Process that emphasizes continuous improvement of health care provided to the public. What is the 8th step in this 10-step process concerned with?
A. Establishing thresholds for evaluation
B. Collecting and organizing data
C. Initiating evaluation
D. Taking actions to improve care and service

D. is the correct answer.

JCAHO's 10-Step Process:
Step 8. Take actions to improve care and service:
a. Teams recommend and/or take actions.

9.032   JCAHO has a 10-Step Process that emphasizes continuous improvement of health care provided to the public. What is the 9th step in this 10-step process concerned with?
A. Assessing the effectiveness of actions and maintaining the gain
B. Communicating results to relevant individuals and groups
C. Maintaining a written log of all changes and outcomes
D. Publishing all findings connected with improvements

A. is the correct answer.

JCAHO's 10-Step Process:
Step 9. Assess the effectiveness of actions and maintain the gain:
a. Assess to determine whether care and service have improved;
b. If not, further action is determined;
c. (a) and (b) are repeated until improvement is achieved and maintained;
d. Monitoring is maintained and priorities for monitoring and the indicators are periodically reassessed.

9.033   JCAHO has a 10-Step Process that emphasizes continuous improvement of health care provided to the public. What is the 10th step in this 10-step process concerned with?
A. Assessing the effectiveness of actions and maintaining the gain
B. Communicating results to relevant individuals and groups
C. Maintaining a written log of all changes and outcomes
D. Publishing all findings connected with improvements

B. is the correct answer.

JCAHO's 10-Step Process:
Step 10. Communicate results to relevant individuals and groups:
a. Teams forward conclusion, actions and results to leaders and to relevant individuals, committees, departments and services;
b. Disseminate information as necessary;
c. Leaders and others receive and disseminate comments, reactions and information from involved individuals and groups (see Bibliography).

9.034   The Microbiology department is concerned that too many of the specimens collected for blood cultures are contaminated with skin flora. For the next 30 days, the Microbiology department is going to compile information concerning specimens drawn for blood cultures. The data to be collected include the total number of specimens drawn for this test, the total number of false positives due to skin contaminants, the locations of the patients with false-positive results, the time and the shift during which the false positives were drawn, and the individual who drew the sample. At this point forward, which steps of JCAHO's 10-Step Process for Quality Assessment will be applied to a situation that needs improvement?
A. The entire JCAHO 10-Step Process
B. Steps 1–5
C. Steps 6–10
D. JCAHO's 10-Step Process does not apply

C. is the correct answer.

For the Microbiology department to be concerned about the number of false-positive blood cultures being collected, the 5th step of JCAHO's process must have been violated. Now that the Microbiology department has been alerted, it is going to institute the 6th to the 10th steps of the 10-step process. Scanning monitors already in place have alerted the department to a possible problem. Focused monitors are now going to be employed to provide data concerning the problem. After the data have been collected, they will be evaluated. The percentage of false positives will be compared to a standard of acceptability; there will be an attempt to note trends that might pinpoint a particular time, area or individual that is contributing to an unacceptable trend. If appropriate, corrective action will be implemented and then the corrective action will have to be monitored to determine its effectiveness. Finally, the Microbiology department must share its findings with all pertinent personnel so that improvement can be effected.

Bibliography

Joint Commission on Accreditation of Healthcare Organizations. *Transitions: From QA to CQI: Using CQI Approaches to Monitor, Evaluate, and Improve Quality*. Oakbrook Terrace, IL: JCAHO, 1991

http://ccme-mac4.bsd.uchicago.eduCCMPolicies/Hosp/AHAbillrts

NCCLS Specimen Collection. *Procedure for the Collection of Diagnostic Blood Specimens by Venipuncture*. NCCLS Document H3-A3, Vol. 11, No. 10, July 1991